Neuropathy

Conditions of Nerve Pain and Dysfunction

(Get Rid of Diabetic Neuropathy and Get Your Life Back)

Donald Vibbert

Published By **Phil Dawson**

Donald Vibbert

Neuropathy: Conditions of Nerve Pain and Dysfunction (Get Rid of Diabetic Neuropathy and Get Your Life Back)

ISBN   978-1-998038-57-2

Legal & Disclaimer

The information contained in this book is not designed to replace or take the place of any form of medicine or professional medical advice. The information in this book has been provided for educational & entertainment purposes only.

The information contained in this book has been compiled from sources deemed reliable, and it is accurate to the best of the Author's knowledge; however, the Author cannot guarantee its accuracy and validity and cannot be held liable for any errors or omissions. Changes are periodically made to this book. You must consult your doctor or get professional medical advice before using any of the suggested remedies, techniques, or information in this book.

Table Of Contents

Chapter 1: Pain Self-Assessment

The first step is for determining and managing the discomfort. In order to think like a psychotherapist think about the different ways the pain can affect you and others surrounding you.

In the process of creating a successful treatment plan, you need to incorporate the following elements:

1. Determine the extent of the discomfort.

2. Review the characteristics of signs.

3. Think about your roles in life in your family.

4. Set short-term and longer-term objectives.

5. Choose the best method for reducing the pain.

6. Create a plan of action and then modify it as needed.

7. Write down your accomplishments.

Through any treatment course, it is important to improve your knowledge and be confident that the effort you put into it will result in positive outcomes. Additionally, you must examine the extent of your discomfort consistently.

Reporting and explaining the pain you experience is among the very first questions that therapists is likely to ask you during your initial assessment. A lot of times, when therapists assess children, teens as well as seniors, they realize the symptoms of pain don't always reflect the exact symptoms For instance:

Children and teens can are unable to articulate certain pain-related symptoms (such as numbness and tingling). If they are unable to express clearly what they're experiencing, pain signs are often misunderstood or treated in a wrong way.

The elderly are often under-reporting or not revealing their pain levels in any way. Some will tell you, "the pain is no big deal, I'm old and it's just my arthritis acting up". The truth is, a rise in old age doesn't necessarily translate to that there is a rise in the pain. In any examination, senior citizens are required to report precisely what they feel.

Although methods of describing discomfort vary, it's usually done numerically, using the scale of 0-10 (0=No Pain, 10=The Most pain). If your pain is at a level of 10 or more, a therapist may recommend urgent medical treatment. This image illustrates an average pain scale.

Levels of pain are subjective, only the person who feels the pain can decide on the degree of pain. Two individuals with similar injury often experience different degrees of pain because of different levels of tolerance.

If the patient is child who is non-verbal, cognitively impaired or a child the therapist may utilize an instrument for pain that puts an emphasis on facial expressions as opposed to an actual numerical scale. The Wong-Baker Pain Rating Scale permits anyone who has been struggling to look at the facial expression that is most appropriate to describe what the person is feeling. Whatever the situation an assessment of their own pain is an excellent starting point that should never be missed.

Following is a 3-page assessment tool for pain designed to aid in keeping your on the right track with your treatment plan. The tool is intended to serve to guide you, since it permits you to write your personal experiences.

It is a Pain Self-Assessment tool is not restricted to the initial process and is intended to be utilized throughout the therapy process, as a instrument for measuring.

Once you've rated your degree of pain, you can think about the features. While in a peaceful space at your own home, you can close your eyes. Then try to comprehend how your sensations feel, such as:

- Does the area of pain appear cold or warm in the area of contact?

Do you experience the sensation of tingling?

Do you feel a pain or sharpness around the site of pain?

Do you feel tension or heaviness?

Are there any pouding or feeling of throbbing?

Are there any numbness, or pain-like sensations at the location?

Examining the specific features of pain will help you decide on the ideal approach to treatment. This Pain Self Assessmet Tool will give you a framework throughout the procedure.

PAIN SELF-ASSESSMENT TOOL

ASK YOURSELF THESE QUESTIONS:

1. What is my pain number on an scale from 0 to 10? (0=no pain, 10=very severe pain) I would like to know:

2. What would you describe as characteristic pain (i.e. sharp, dull, aching, sore, tingling):

_____

3. What increases the pain level:

_____

4. What decreases the pain level:

_____

REFLECT ON DAILY ROLES & RESPONSIBILITIES THAT ARE NEGATIVELY IMPACTED BY PAIN:

Priority #1:

_____

_____

Priority #2:

_____

_____

Priority #3:

_____

_____

SETTING GOALS:

1. In the short-term, my goal is to decrease my level of pain by: _____

In this particular number of weeks/days In this example:

2. My Personal Short-Term Goal:

_____

_____

_____

For this amount of days/weeks In this example:

1. In the long run, my goal is to decrease my number of painful episodes by: _____

In this particular number of months/weeks Within this number of weeks/months:

_____

2. My Personal Long-Term Goal:

_____

_____

_____

For this amount of days/weeks Within this number of days/weeks: _____

A LIST OF THINGS TO DO FOR DECREASING PAIN (Check the items that are applicable):

___Stretch ___Exercise ___Activities ___Soak

___Elevate ___Rest ___Ice ___Heat

___Educate on Injury/Disease ___Meditate

___Postural Training ___Massage ___Kinesio Taping

___Yoga/Tai Chi ___Counselling

Contact an Support Group

___Other_____

_____

DETAIL YOUR PLAN TO ACHIEVE YOUR GOALS:

1. This is what I'm going to do:

_____

_____

_____

_____

What is the number of hours/days you work:

_____

2. This is what I'm going to do:

_____

_____

_____

_____

What is the number of hours/days you work:

_____

_____

3. I'll do this:

_____

_____

_____

_____

The number of hours/days that you can work in:

JOURNAL YOUR RESULTS:

_____

_____

_____

_____

_____

_____

_____

_____

Chapter 2: Acute -Vs- Chronic Pain

What exactly is acute pain? It is a pain that occurs following an injury, or results from an illness that has been diagnosed recently or illness.

The typical symptoms of acute pain may differ, but typically include intense, painful and throbbing the sensation of pounding. The symptoms of acute pain can stem from the following factors:

* A broken bone or sprain

* A burn or cut

* A strain or muscle pull

* Headaches

* A dental or medical procedure

Menstrual cramps every month

* Delivery and labor of a child

The initial pain stage can be quite short and lasts anywhere from a minute to 12 weeks. The immediate sensation may be described as light, moderate or intense. The first sign of an acute wound may be soft and pink, or swollen or swollen.

The mild acute pain is effectively treated with a proper program and with little intervention. But, excessive to extreme acute pain may cause significant life changes, requiring you to change your daily routine. Lifestyle, routines and financial situation are a major concern in the event of persistent moderate acute pain.

Acute pain that is severe may be mentally, physically as well as emotionally crippling. In addition, changes in behavior and stress from acute pain may affect the relationships you have with your loved ones. There is a silver lining in any degree of acute pain is that it will last less than twelve weeks. If it lasts over that period it's classed as chronic suffering.

What is Chronic Pain? Chronic pain can last many years and requires a lengthy dedication and a strict constantly changing plan for managing the symptoms.

The most common symptoms that are characteristic of chronic pain are defined as but not restricted to, aching burning, numbness, and tingling sensations. Commonly, the causes and illnesses that contribute to chronic pain can include:

* Arthritis

* Fibromyalgia

* Cancer

* Neuropathy

* Sciatic nerve disorders

* Headaches and migraines.

* Myofascial soft tissue disorder

Chronic pain has a significant impact on the your quality of life in nearly everything, from financial stability and ability to work in a professional setting, through personal relationships as well as the duration of one's own life. If not treated properly chronic pain may result in the use of prescription painkillers or prescription opioids.

Once you begin to be a therapist, you can think about using a range of methods for relieving pain. The next chapters will provide a range of methods that you could select from. However, first, the table provides a summary of the distinction between chronic and acute pain with the intention of clarifying the differences.

Chapter 3: Techniques For Acute Pain Relief

Each person responds differently and cold therapies for immediate pain relief. Certain people prefer warmth to relax joints and muscles, while some prefer cold in order to soothe the painful area.

One of the most commonly requested questions from Therapists is "When do I use a hot pack versus a cold pack for pain relief?" A therapist's perspective, it's straightforward to answer since therapy professionals think about more than just discomfort. Consider the advantages that cold or hot treatments can bring like:

1. If there's swelling, the application of cold therapy are not only able to reduce the pain through stimulating or numbing painful area, but they may also prevent bleeding from occurring or reduce the circulation of blood.

2. If you're experiencing pain and pain, but little or no swelling, then heat treatments can

be calming and relax the tissues. This can ease joint stiffness and increase the flexibility.

Prior to applying hot and cold treatments, therapists assess the condition of the skin, by evaluating it the skin for warmth, tightness or a cooling sensation. Therapists also will determine the presence of any signs of skin coloration (i.e. either red or blue) at or around the site of pain.

Making Your Own Cold Pack

If you slip and injure your ankle, the majority of us are familiar with applying an ice-cold compress immediately following the incident. However, many don't be aware of the reasons why they should apply the compression.

Therapists understand that one of the advantages of applying a cold wrap during an accident is that it will reduce or stop the flow of blood to stop excessive bleeding. Cold packs are commonly used for numbing the region of injury as well as reducing swelling.

Cold packs may be stimulating and can stimulate joints and muscles. But, it is not recommended to apply cold compresses to injuries longer than 15 to 10 minutes. It is an excellent practice to do at the home environment as well.

In the event of applying cold packs in your home, observe the color of your skin and its integrity throughout the application to make sure you don't notice any changes.

The "ziploc gel cold pack" can be made in the your home. It is a similar gel-pack as one that is used in therapeutic facilities. Ingredients and the steps required to make your own cold packs include:

* 2 ziploc bags

1 cup water

* 1 cup of ruby alcohol

Blue dye can be used in lieu

Step 1. Double the Ziploc bag to limit the chance of leakage.

Step 2. Include 1 cup water along with 1/2 cup of ruby alcohol (double the amount above to make more large chill packs).

Step 3: Put the bag inside the freezer for around one hour or until the packing feels soft and gel-like (not too stiff or hard) to allow for better contouring of the area of injury.

Step 4: After applying the cold compress on the area of pain It is always advisable to use a cloth between your body and bag.

If you are still experiencing pain, but the swelling has diminished, within the period of 48 hours, a therapist might look into a hot-pack to treat a fresh injury, in order to increase blood flow to the site to aid in the healing process and decrease the pain.

Making Your Own Hot Pack

Most often, therapists employ hot packs to reduce the intensity of pain. They also improve blood flow and reduce muscle tightness to allow you to participate with activities and exercises. Heating aids in bringing fresh oxygenated blood flow to the area of pain to assist in the process of healing.

Therapists should not apply heat packs when there's evidence of severe to moderate swelling. Instead, they employ cold compresses. It is advisable not to apply an ice or hot pack on the area of pain for a maximum of 15 minutes Always use an obstruction such as towels between it to the surface. After that, you should monitor your area of the skin during the treatment.

The components needed to create the moist heat packs at home include:

* A thick sports socks or 10"x10" rectangular piece of fabric, such as an afghan

Needle and thread are needed to sew

* 4-6 cups uncooked white rice that is dry and uncooked

* Aromatherapy items (optional)

Step 1: Place the non-cooked ingredients to the sock or into the middle of the scarf.

Step 2: If you wish, use aromatherapy products, like lavender or peppermint oils.

Step 3. Tie or stitch into the sock by using a needle and thread.

Step 4. Microwave for about three minutes. The hot packs should remain in the warm position for about 20 mins.

In the outpatient clinic the level of pain you report will determine the best treatment. The therapists treat minor acute pain in a different way than the moderate or severe type of painful. Examples:

If you are experiencing minor acute discomfort (ranging between 1-3 of 10) the therapist might use physical activity and exercise during treatment sessions as in the event that they're properly checked.

If you are experiencing intense to moderate acute discomfort that is between 4 and 10 in 10, the treatment process will generally begin with a cold or hot compress, followed by mild stretching and massage. In the next step, muscle therapy like compression bandaging, or kinesiotaping is utilized prior to lower-impact activities and workouts.

* Therapists can employ an array of both treatments that are cold and hot when severe pain is present with significant swelling. Combining extreme cold and hot temperatures is called"contrast bath. "contrast bath".

What is a Contrast Bath?

A contrast bath involves an exercise that involves alternating cool and hot temperatures for the purpose of creating an action of natural pumping (called vasodilation and vasoconstriction) in order to reduce the swelling.

If you are experiencing mild or extreme swelling that is like it is throbbing, tight, and aching, then it is possible that your swelling could be exacerbating the pain symptoms. Contrast baths are fast and only lasts about 10 minutes.

The contrast bath may be done by immersing the entire area of pain with alternating cold and hot soaks or alternately applying the cold and hot packs directly over the area of pain (with an insulating cloth to avoid burning) over a period of approximately 10 minutes.

The process begins by distributing two minutes of hot water, after which you can apply 1 minute cold. Repeat the procedure to complete 10 minutes. In general, when you take in a contrast bath, the temperature of temperature of the hot water shouldn't exceed the temperature of 104° F (40 degrees Celsius) while cold water must stay between 45 and 70 ° F (7 between 21 and 70 degrees Celsius).

Make sure to follow the contrast bath by self-massaging as well as KT tapping to help relieve pain. Some helpful tips are listed below for your convenience in your home.

What is Self-Massaging?

Self-massage is a simple and effective way to ease your pain and relieve the tightness in your muscles as well as trigger points (also known as knots which may feel on the skin).

Self-massaging releases the endorphins which naturally relieve pain. The practice of self-massage can be done at home. It can then be integrated into any treatment plan to ease pain.

Basic Tips for Self-Massaging:

Tip #1. Lay down or sit in a comfortable place.

Tip #2. Relax; do your best not to be stressed.

Tip #3: If the skin appears dry, apply creams or lotions that do not cause irritation to the skin, however will help in gliding over the skin.

TIP #4 If you are applying compression, begin with gentle increasing the pressure gradually.

Tips #5 Start with small thumb-circles on or around the area of pain. Begin with the fingers instead of your entire hand, will help determine the exact location where pain is situated and the intensity of it.

Tips #6 Adjust the angle of your hand using your hands into a fist with your palm or the open-hand method.

Tip #7 Start making longer strokes, not circles, by moving them horizontally as well as vertically.

Tips #8: During self-massage, lengthen and reduce the length of your muscles by stretching and then repositioning your body.

TIP #9 Try other methods at or near the painful location, like gently tap, shaking, and spreading the skin.

What is Kinesio Taping?

Kinesio tapping, also referred to by the name of KT tape is well-liked in rehabilitation facilities. It's often used by people who play sports and take part in everyday activities since it offers quick relief from pain.

The relief, however, tends to be short-lived and requires practice to properly apply the tape. The book gives you basic information on the advantages of KT tape as well with helpful advice on how to apply it.

Making your own skills perfect using KT tape is a process that requires time and perseverance. Your goal is to discover an appropriate level of "pull" on the skin which the tape could offer, to provide relief for pain. It is possible that you will need to observe on your own how KT tape is used on other people, in order to learn more about different techniques that could be employed.

The tape consists of spandex, cotton spandex, cotton and adhesive. Once it is applied, it permits you to engage in of your range of motion activities as well as exercises. A brief overview of the advantages of KT tape, when applied correctly is as follows:

* Help improve circulation and speed healing.

* Reducing discomfort

* Provide joint and muscle support

* Reduce swelling

How to use Self-kinesio Taping

TIP #1 Preparing the skin surrounding the painful area by cleansing it and removing any lotions, or liquid substances, then shaving it off if there's an abundance of hair around the location.

Tip #2 Cut and square around the corners of the tape to avoid catching onto clothes.

Tip #3 Use KT tape 45-60 mins prior to exercising or exercise

Tips #4 There are four different types of KT applications.

* No stretch

* Light stretch

* Moderate stretch

* Heavy stretch

In order to relieve pain, the majority KT tapes are applied using moderate or light stretching.

Tips #5 Don't touch the adhesive tape. This can cause overlapping as well as excessive wear on the tape.

TIP #6 Frequent skin check-ups is important to avoid irritation. Be aware of skin redness and itching.

Tip #7 Don't become obsessed because the skin needs to breathe! KT tape must be left in place for no more than one up to two days.

If KT tape doesn't help reduce acute pain and swelling, you should think like an Occupational Therapist to combat the signs of acute pain and swelling with the RICE technique that stands for:

* Rest

* Ice

* Compression

* Elevation

The RICE Method is utilized for treating acute bruises or sprains. It also helps with injured soft tissue, as well as signs of neurological diseases including stroke Alzheimer's, Multiple Sclerosis and Parkinson's Disease.

What are the reasons therapists employ RICE? RICE Method?

Therapists utilize the RICE method due to its ability to strengthen muscles and bones immediately after you experience symptoms due to an illness or injury. Additionally, the method using ice, rest compressing, elevation, and rest helps to stop swelling excessively and recurring bleeding. It also aids in faster healing.

Therapists are aware that the four components (rest in the form of ice, rest, elevation and compression) have a crucial role in rehabilitation and recovery.

Relaxing the site of pain is crucial since in order for it to heal it is important to take a break from lifting weights for a while. Use this time to relax take advantage of it to establish the best way to control the intensity of your pain. Take a look at meditation or deep breathing as an alternative to medications.

Ice is crucial as it reduces the bleeding as well as numbs discomfort in injuries that are acute. The swelling that occurs in these injuries can cause acute pain, which is which is characterized as heavy and tight.

Compression, the final component in RICE, concentrates on providing support and relief. Elastic bandages like Ace wraps may be utilized however, they must be applied with care so that there is no disruption to blood circulation.

Elevation is the last element. It's crucial because it permits fluids and blood to flow in a natural direction towards the heart. So, you should place your body part at least 6 to 10 inches over the heart, if you can. There is a possibility of lying down.

Acute Muscle Pain

Muscle pain can also be referred to as myalgia in the eyes of therapy professionals. The most common causes of muscular pain are tension and tension. They can also be caused by sprains, strains, injury to the tissue or adverse consequences of medication.

The causes of chronic muscle pain can be different. It could be a symptom of a disease, infection or medical issue that is more detailed in the following chapter.

The pain of a muscle is typically specific, with the symptoms being experienced in only a few muscles, not spread over the entire body. Muscle pain that is acute is often intense, and can be accompanied by symptoms that range from cramping, burning and stabbing pains, to discomfort and pain.

If you begin to think like a professional and therapist, your acute muscle pain relief must include some methods that were previously discussed in previous chapters, including:

- self-massaging

- KT tape

Hot and cold packs applications

If you are looking to reduce the time between painful muscle spasms, the consistency of your approach is essential. This is a suggested routine to reduce the intensity of muscle pain

A Suggested Daily Plan for Acute Muscle Pain:

In the morning, while lying you are in bed, lie on your back, and move all the areas of your body to the max of your ability. As if your whole body is being a "log" is a good option when rolling from the across the right and left sides of the bed to ensure that you can roll like a whole.

Begin your day with or soaking in warm water or a hot wrap for 5 minutes (if there's not any swelling) to ensure adequate blood flow. At night, you may change to an ice pack should you wish to.

A gentle compressing of the muscles that are aching with a gentle stretch (ACE) wraps can offer the relief needed and support for muscles all whole day.

Afternoon: Massage your area for about 10-15 minutes.

Strategies for massaging muscles

Tips #1 Warming oils can be soothing to muscles and can provide further pain relief. But, you should apply the warm oil to first your palm and do not apply directly onto the body.

Tips #2: Begin to massage superficially (on the surface on the face) prior to advancing as well as moving to move away from pain sites before moving towards it.

TIP #3 Use strokes that start beginning at the base of your thumb, along the tips of your fingers for 2-3, and the bottom of your small finger if you're looking to get deeper into or focus on small, specific regions.

It's the perfect opportunity when you can apply KT tape or some light compression bandaging at the location. The best option is to alternate the two to stay clear of using KT tape on a daily basis.

Perform postural exercise along with other gentle exercises, such as the ones described in chapter 6.

Relaxation and rest is essential at the end of the day. Take an energizing bath.

Baths with contrast can be calming. This technique was explained earlier in this chapter. It lets the body naturally eliminate excess fluid. When contrast baths are conducted properly, they allow for improved functionality and comfort for people who is suffering from pain.

Acute Bone & Joint Pain

The treatment of acute joint and bone discomfort is similar to the treatment of muscular discomfort. The bruising, fractured or cracking of a bone, cancer of the bone or joint inflammation due to arthritis may cause extreme discomfort and even debilitation.

Common areas for joint pain comprise, but aren't restricted to shoulder, hands or knees. They can also affect ankles, knees and the ankles. The site of pain may feel hot to the touch, with tension and heaviness in the region of the.

The typical symptoms can vary between a sensation of irritation to sharpness in bones and joints. The pain may be recurrent all day long, spreading between joints.

An everyday routine can help to reduce pain, to allow you to continue to work productively. Here is the daily schedule to help ease pain:

A Suggested Daily Plan for Acute Bone & Joint Pain

Morning: Prior to rising and stepping out of bed do some stretching exercises. It's the best position that to be in. When you're in bed, move your body on both side of your bed concentrate on lengthening and reducing your muscles to ease pain from joints and bones that they serve.

If there's none (or slight) swelling, apply an ice pack for a period of 5-10 minutes in order to increase circulation into the joint. In the case of severe swelling or excessive you can apply a cold compress for between 5 and 10 minutes instead. It is also possible to alternate cold and hot packs over a period that lasts 10 minutes (2 minute of warm and 1 minute cold) that is called the contrast bath.

After you have gotten off the bed, you can apply additional gentle stretching for about 15 minutes either standing or sitting following application of cold or hot packs.

Afternoon: Massage gently the site of pain using or without lotions, creams or oils that warm.

An area that is larger will necessitate an open-hand method and rolling the palms using a light, smooth compression of the pain area.

* To relieve pain between joints, apply pressure with fingers with tips that are about 2 or 3 inches to get deeper as needed.

Participate in a proper exercise routine for your postural (techniques to improve postural posture are described in Chapter 6.). Be sure to employ the correct body mechanics for everyday activities, and to use proper ergonomics when sitting for long periods of time. Practice sitting on your back in an office chair, so that your spine stays in alignment.

The evening: Use evening: Apply the RICE procedure at the close of your day. Rest your joints and bones and ice them if there is swelling. If it persists and apply compression (before getting ready to go to sleep) before elevating the knee if needed.

It is important to keep in mind that pain in the acute stage, be it bone or muscular, could develop into chronic, long-lasting suffering over the course of twelve months. Particularly, when a person is unable to take care of the pain properly.

Chapter 4: Techniques For Chronic Pain Relief

Chronic pain is often hard to manage, and while it's usually not risky, it may change your life. Similar to the relief of acute pain it is recommended to perform a series of range-of motion and stretching exercises in conjunction regularly massaging the area of pain are excellent ways to ease the pain that is chronic.

Since chronic pain can last for years, it could begin to affect the person's mental or emotional health. Consider regular sessions of meditation and counseling in order to reduce anxiety, depression and stress. Numerous people opt for yoga and Tai Chi classes for relaxing and to ease anxiety.

Additionally, it's crucial to implement lifestyle modifications to reduce discomfort and maintain it to the level that is manageable which is two out of 10. A few lifestyle modifications might be worth considering are postural exercises, changing your diet, and using proper movements for your body during daily activities.

There are a variety of ailments and conditions that cause chronic pain. However, this section will concentrate on three diagnoses that are common that include:

* Arthritis

* Peripheral neuropathy

* Myofascial disorders

Each of these causes constant pain in the small joints, the larger muscles and bones. Together or in isolation, they may be debilitating for an individual as well as last for a number of years.

Arthritis and peripheral neuropathy as well as myofascial diseases are wonderful cases to explore in this book since they all have characteristics of pain like other chronic illnesses including stroke, cancer and heart diseases, diabetes as well as neurological diseases and other.

As you keep reading about peripheral neuropathy, arthritis and myofascial issues and peripheral neuropathy, you'll begin to think about the most effective methods to manage the symptoms of pain without looking at the disease itself.

Therapists are educated to take a critical look at the symptoms you experience and the process of disease. But, they also are aware of when they should shift to ensure the most effective outcome.

Arthritis

A lot of people suffer everyday chronic arthritis discomfort. It is a shame that waking up in the morning and then going to sleep suffering from stiff and painful joints as well as muscles and bones can cause emotional and physical impact. As there's no treatment for arthritis, sufferers are usually left having to learn how to deal with the discomfort.

What is Arthritis?

The most frequent forms are osteoarthritis and rheumatoid. Other types of illnesses can cause arthritis, or exhibit arthritis-like symptoms for example:

* Lupus

* Fibromyalgia

* Gout

* Lyme disease

Rheumatoid arthritis (RA) can be found in small joints, like the fingers, when your immune system attack the joint's lining and makes it more difficult to grasp and pin objects. RA may also change the structure and form of the joint. This can result in visible swelling of the knuckles as well as other hand/fingers deformities.

Osteoarthritis (OA) is a condition that occurs within the joint at the end of a bigger bone (such as the knee). The condition can progress to chronic extreme pain when you place loads on the knee joint during the course of your day.

OA may also cause damage to cartilage until it is now possible to walk and sitting bone-on-bone. In many cases, severe and chronic suffering due to OA causes debility and reduced range of motion.

Arthritis Pain Relief Techniques

The most effective pain-relief treatment for arthritis differs for each person. Certain people favor heat instead of cold to ease pain while others favor lowintensity exercises over vigorous ones for joint flexibility.

Stretching towels, which are carried out at home, is an excellent way to increase performance and ease pain for patients suffering from arthritis.

The other common methods for pain relief in arthritis are however, they aren't limited to:

* Compression socks or gloves

Hot or cold packs

Gentle massage strokes onto the area of pain.

* Stretching exercises like yoga or tai-chi

Chronic pain can last for a long time as it gets worse, so over time it is possible to think about mobile devices and other machines to provide comfort at home, for example:

Outpatient therapy facilities foam body rollers, and paraffin devices have been proven to be effective in helping with pain when they are used properly. They are extremely effective when used at home when used in conjunction with everyday workouts to ease the pain of inflammation and muscle tightness.

Arthritis is an joint disorder that is inflammatory and can be seen in a sporadic manner. Apart from the massage equipment and other ways that could be utilized to obtain relief from arthritis as well as other diagnoses similar to it.

Certain foods, for instance, contain antioxidants and vitamins as well as help to reduce discomfort you feel as a result of cancer, diabetes or heart diseases. Here are a few examples below:

* Ginger and Turmeric can reduce the inflammation that is caused by arthritis, boost digestive health and improve digestion and acts as an anti-inflammatory non-steroidal drug to ease menstrual discomfort in women. It also helps reduce the painful signs associated with Crohn's Disease IBS, stomach ulcers, and inflammation resulting from surgery post-surgery.

* Yams and potato are rich in nutrients and fiber as well as a great source of energy that can boost your immune system. They also help in reducing excess fluid that could cause chronic pain. They can alleviate menopausal pain as well as possess anti-cancer properties that help ease discomfort when inflammation develops.

* Omega-3 fish oil can reduce the risk of suffering from heart diseases, boost cholesterol levels, lower blood pressure, and

reduce plaque buildup in arteries. since fish oils possess anti-inflammatory properties, they are able to decrease bone and joint pain as well as stiffness. They also reduce the amount of medication demands for those suffering from arthritis.

Some other popular food items which are rich in Omega-3 and packed with ingredients to fight the painful signs of illness include but are not only, the following:

1. Cod liver oil

2. Walnuts

3. Soy beans

4. Anchovies

5. Chia and flax seeds

Food choices that are healthy and nutritious can not be the sole solution for chronic pain relief. Over the past several centuries the people of all ages have grown cannabis plants in their personal backyards for therapeutic purposes.

While products that contain cannibis (such as CBD oil) remain banned in certain nations, studies conducted in clinical trials have been proving positive regarding the advantages of these supplements to aid in the relief of pain.

The research on the cannabis industry has revealed two major chemical compounds called CBD as well as THC. CBD (used mostly for medical reasons) helps in relaxing you to sleep and offers pain relief. However, THC (primarily used for recreation purposes) can be described as the chemical component which is the ingredient that gives you a intoxicated.

The products of medicinal cannabis tend to be high in CBD and have a low amount of THC.

Cannabis products for recreational use generally contain high levels of THC as well as low in CBD

A Suggested Daily Plan for Relief of Arthritis:

The morning before taking a bath move your body and stretch it with a relaxed state for between 10 and 15 minutes.

Then, if you suffer from an ongoing pain issue in the larger bones (knees or hips) or larger surface regions like your back, sit on the floor using the help of a body roller made from foam or even a towel folded into the form of a log.

* Place your body on top of the roller and support it with a body weight.

• Gently move the area (back and forward) to ensure that the piece lies on the surface of pain.

In the afternoon, apply a hot pack for 5-10 minutes to improve blood flow to the. If you notice moderate to significant swelling, you can apply a cold compress.

The next step is to engage in range of motion or stretching exercises, whether either sitting or standing.

Close your eyes and focus on doing slow stretching exercises until you feel comfortable "end-feel" or when movements get too painful and tight to move further.

The evening: Epsom salt soaks help in relieving pain prior to going to bed because of the magnesium levels. There are many people who use Epsom salt to relieve joint pain or peripheral neuropathy symptoms that can manifest as sensations of tingling or sharp needles and pins on the feet or hands.

Arthritis pain is distinct from the discomfort that peripheral neuropathy sufferers experience. The pleasure of an Epsom salt bath might not suffice. So, you could require an array of methods to get the relief you need from pain.

Peripheral Neuropathy

The peripheral neuropathy may become to be so serious that it can lead to hypersensitivity or numbness to the touch of your body. Many suffer from persistent sensations that are sharp as pins and needles as well as the feeling of cold and hot temperatures that cause discomfort to their body every day.

What is Peripheral Neuropathy?

The word "neuropathy" is familiar to numerous people, particularly patients as having diabetes, lupus, or who are undergoing chemotherapy and radiation treatment. Neuropathy often referred to as neuropathy by many doctors are further explained in the chapter 5.

Peripheral nerve fibers run throughout the body and transmit signals from your brain to organs, and even your extremities like fingers, feet, toes and fingers.

Consider it like multiple cords of cable that run from a single cable box and out into various places in your home. A damaged cable (or an inoperable cable box) is able to interfere with the normal functioning.

The simplest way to describe it is that nerve pain caused by peripheral neuropathy results from the pressure, damage or infection of some or all of the nerves within the body. The disruption in nerve function can result in chronic discomfort if it is not addressed properly. There are more than 100 different types that are peripheral neuropathy-related, the main causes that of the many U.S. therapists hear about is diabetes.

The signs and symptoms of peripheral neuropathy can range in intensity from tingling stabbing and burning to total feeling of numbness or tingling in your feet or hands. There are also quick flashes of hot or cold skin. The symptoms can be repeated and take time to treat properly.

Peripheral Neuropathy Pain Relief Techniques

The technique known as sensory Re-education can be used to aid in de-sensitization of the skin in order to lessen the pain of neuropathy by activating the pathways to sensory that have been affected by disease or injury.

The reason therapists utilize strategies for sensory re-education? Since sensory re-education can be an opportunity to train the brain to experience the sensations it used to feel within the extremities. In theory, through repetition, you're teaching and the brain to react appropriately to damaged nerves.

These home-based strategies for improving your sensory awareness are used by many therapeutic facilities to help educate your nerves' sensory systems to the normal sensations of touch.

Rub different textures across the skin and varying the amount of pressure. Begin by rubbing soft skin textures before moving to rougher skin.

With your eyes closed, attempt to discern the distinction in the texture. Examples of things at home you could utilize include cotton balls Velcro, sandpaper, and tissue.

* Pour 5 cups of cooked rice or beans into an empty bowl. Include small items such as

coins, hair beads or even paper clips. Utilize the affected part to mix the beans or rice by removing and labeling tiny objects, and not having to look.

Variation in temperature, through taking a bath to separate the feeling of the skin. Take a sponge and soak it and hot water. The temperature should not be more than 104 degrees F (40 degrees Celsius). Next, you will squeeze and then release the ball or sponge into warm water for about 10 to 15 minutes. Reverse the process with cold water, with temperatures remaining between 45 and 70 ° F (7 up to 21 ° C).

Use different temperatures by the help with a towel rather than getting your skin soaked.

In other words, let an individual randomly switch between placing an icy and hot towel across your limbs. You must then shut your eyes your temperature and grade it as moderate, mild or even severe.

* The same principle used in varying temperatures could be utilized to determine the presence of touch at an area at the extremity of your body.

As an example, if you close your eyes, and allowing a person to contact a specific part of your body, your task is to determine which body part they have actually touched with the pressure or touch.

Because neuropathy results from nerve injury It is possible to find organic ways to reduce pain and aid in healing. Consider altering your diet so that you include specific foods rich of antioxidants, mineral, and vitamins can aid in fighting the neuropathies and heal nerves such as:

* Consumption and consumption of different fruit, such as blueberries cherries, citrus as well as blackberries and grapes.

* Ingestion of various vegetable including spinach, kale broccoli, brussel sprouts and kale

* Ingestion of various beans, such as black beans, pinto beans, beans from lima as well as lentils

A Suggested Daily Plan for Relief of Neuropathy

The morning: Begin your day by taking a different bath. Alternate soaks of cold and hot water for 10 minutes for your feet or hands.

Afternoon: Rub and rub strokes of various kinds of texture along the lower and upper extremities of your body to help re-educate your sensory system as explained in the previous chapter.

Bring blood to your body through a variety-of-motion workout by pressing and then releasing an kitchen sponge or a hand towel. The exercises for range-of-motion can be completed either in warm and cold water, while extensing and stretching your arms.

In the evening, gently massage your feet and hands in the evening following a tiring day. It is the perfect occasion to make use of your favourite gel or cream or apply a topical medicine that can aid in relieving nerve pain.

A different method of re-education for the senses can be used prior to going to bed. Like we have discussed earlier in this chapter, you can use a huge bowl of beans or rice.

* If you place your feet or your hands into the bowl of beans or rice and beans, you should be able to tell whether it is warm or cold.

If you place your hands inside the bowl, you can see the pieces of each by pressing the pieces one at a time using varying force.

If you imagine yourself as the therapist you're thinking of, you'll know the neuropathy could persist for many several months. Understanding how to treat the symptoms as early as possible is essential. One of the best aspects with the neuropathy that is it typically remains at the upper and lower extremities, in contrast to myofascial conditions.

Myofascial Disorder

Though it's not well-known to the majority of people Myofascial pain can cause more severe pain than neuropathy in the peripheral. Myofascial discomfort is experienced throughout the body, such as your back and shoulders, maybe radiating out to other places such as your neck.

Myofascial symptoms may persist for a long time (especially in the case of another neurological condition like Parkinson's or Multiple Sclerosis). Myofascial pain may cause anxiety, insomnia as well as a limited range of motion in the body. All of which can affect the quality of your living.

What is Myofascial?

Myofascial refers to the layer of connective tissue that surrounds and supports the organs, muscles as well as bones of your body. It is composed of water, collagen, as well as cells that help in the proper functioning.

A simple, but graphic way to see myofascia is by laying down an rib-slice of raw meat prior to roasting, grilling, or baking. The white (and occasionally transparent) sheet that connects between the bones and meat is a symbol of the support and security of the structures. Its secure attachment to the bone and the meat is difficult to consume this is one reason are advised to decide to remove it.

Myofascial tissue fibers function in a similar way inside your body. They maintain the structure of our muscles as well as the flexibility. They keep the bone, organs and tissues together and working as a piece. But, it could become too tight, or even injured, which can cause extreme discomfort in our bodies.

The two most common causes of myofascial discomfort:

1. Myofascial muscle tissue that is stretched out too tight through activities, exercise or performing improper physique mechanics.

2. The source of the "trigger point" (commonly referred to as a knot) under the myofascial muscle.

Common causes may result in large areas of pain which could eventually develop sensitivity to the touch of your hand. This may initially manifest as a nagging pain, but it is more often a sign of persistent permanent suffering. The goal of this kind of pain relieving is to attain the "act of release" or sometimes referred to as "myofascial release".

What is myofascial relaxation? It is a method to relieve the muscle tension or to massage away knots until there is a real physical and emotional change. This technique has been studied extensively by certified massage therapists. Here are six methods that could offer relief from chronic myofascial issues at the ease of the privacy of your own living space.

The first step is to sit or lie to rest in a peaceful area.

Third: Practice the techniques of slow breathing to relax.

Third: Apply a variety of ways to massage your hands or a foam roller cloth or other object to determine your "right pressure" point (only you will be able to identify what is like).

Fourth: Avoid causing cause irritation to the region by applying heavy pressure. If you notice yourself grinning or squinting when you perform myofascial relaxation techniques If you do, it means that excessive pressure has been placed on your body.

Five: Look for "good pain", the one that's tolerable . The good kind of pain will make you think, "oh that's a bit painful but it felt like I needed it!"

Sixth: Decide if each move or stroke has an impact on.

In order to relieve myofascial pain it is important to recognize your personal experiences with painful. Learn to assess it, learn to define the pain, and identify the location of it.

Most importantly, pay attention to the way your hands can provide relief (i.e. the position you are placing your hands in, and how much the pressure they are putting on your hands). Here are some suggestions to assist you.

Tips #1: Assess your level of pain before trying to get rid of it and lessening the trigger points. If you feel it is a extreme pain (in the 9-10 range) after each massage or motion, then rate it once more.

Tip #2: Attempt to lower the tension of your muscles by 1 to 2 pain levels through applying pressure that is the "right pressure" while engaging with self-massage, and by slowing the range of motion. What's the best pressure? It's subjective. That means that only you will know what is as a sense of the relief.

Tips #3: Give yourself some time (at minimum 10 minutes) for you to feel like the muscles relax and physiologically adjusting.

Tip #4: If you spot trigger points or "knots" under your skin You increase your awareness of the degree of pain and the location.

Myofascial Pain Relief Techniques

Four commonly used therapeutic methods for myofascial pain relief you can perform at home include the following:

- Soft log roller

- Foam log roller

Self-massage using household items

Applications for heat

If you are experiencing moderate to extreme myofascial pain, you can make your own log roll using a bath towel or rolls of paper towels.

Bath Towels To create your own lumbar roll take a bath towel, fold it in half and then fold it in two lengthwise and then roll it into. Utilize rubber bands on the towel to hold it rolling up.

Paper Towel roll There's no reason to change or reassemble the whole roll. It can be put in a position and compressed in order to make it more supportive and comfortable to the back of the lumbar spine or other areas that are painful.

If you are experiencing mild pain in your myofascial area you can use a round item like tennis balls, large fruits that you can find in your fridge or even a roll of foam. This can create more tension on the tissues. This could include:

* When using several objects like tennis balls, or fruits (lemon/oranges) Place them inside an sock, and tie knots at the ends. Additionally, make a knot with both objects.

The foam log roller is readily available at many stores. They provide the relief you need, however they tend to be much more rigid than fruit or towel log rollers. This makes them ideal for people with mild pain.

Self-massaging using home products can be extremely helpful in the location and relaxation of tight muscles, and removing trigger areas. Always remember to stay safe and secure.

Place a mat on the floor or put your body against the wall, while sitting. These home furnishings can be used to massage yourself regions that are not within reach of your arms:

- Kitchen rolling pin,

- Broom stick handle

- Frozen water bottle

- Tennis ball

- - Fruit (orange or lemon)

- Paper towel roll

- Pillows

Make use of a tennis ball, or fruit to focus on certain areas that are tender or to trigger points or knots. Below are some steps that will help you understand how to use tiny objects, such as fruits for pain relief.

Step 1: Recall the previous tips to be successful in your exercise, including being relaxed in your breathing, taking proper deep breaths, and noting your level of pain during the entire process.

Step 2: When lying on a mat for a floor or leaning against the wall, set a tennis ball(s) on the wall or floor as well as your trigger point.

Step 3: Roll gently over the object until you are feeling "good" pain, using the pressure to determine the area of discomfort, as you slowly perform rolls.

Step 4: Give yourself between 10-12 strokes or rolls to provide the relief of pain.

Heating applications are another excellent method to ease the chronic pain of myofascial joints. The safest temperature is 90 to 100°F assists in relaxing muscles and can bring fresh blood to the area of pain.

The increase in blood flow through heat (dry or humid) helps the new blood remove waste products of lactic acid, hence decreasing the pain. If you are suffering from persistent pain, a portion of the discomfort is due to the accumulation of ineffective lactic acid.

What exactly is lactic acid waste? It is formed when there is a lack of oxygen within the body's tissues to breakdown glucose (which is necessary to generate energy). The waste is formed in your tissue muscles, and is then transported to the bloodstream.

Examples of applications that are hot can include but not be restricted to:

* Hot pack that's moist (design your personal hot pack following the instructions in chapter 3.)

A hot bath or shower will provide warm humid warmth.

* Hot water bottles that has been heated by the microwave (always covered with a cloth between the bottle and the skin) will provide the warmth of a moist environment

The heating pads of electric offer dry heating

Here are a few tips to assist you in making the right decision about when to choose between moist and dry warmth.

Tips #1: Moist warmth like hot baths and showers are convenient and can provide immediate relief. Furthermore humid heat packs as well as hot water absorb into the skin rapidly and then get into joints and muscles.

But, it's difficult to control the temperature in moist temperatures; and if in a hurry, you may put on excessive heat and harm your skin.

Tip #2 Dry heat, such as heating pads with electric are easily available at local retailers and feature temperatures that can be controlled.

However, heating pads made of electricity are unable to be used with the correct cords which can cause skin to become thirsty.

Be aware of the need to take precautions or stop using heating completely if you notice any of the following symptoms:

* If you've got open bleeding, bruises, or significant swelling.

* If you have diabetes, hypertension or any disease that involves veins and arteries like deep vein the thrombosis (DVT) and peripheral vascular diseases (PVD).

A Suggested Daily Plan for Relief of Myofascial Pain

The morning: Begin your day by relaxing with a method such as meditation or yoga and the right breathing exercises that help reduce tension and stress that has built up within your muscles.

The practice of breathing through the lips can be used safely during the entire day. Here is an example of an breathing method that is effortless to do.

1. In a calm area, you can relax your shoulders and neck.

2. Keep your mouth shut and breathe slowly with your nose, as if you had been smelling roses two to 3 minutes.

3. You can purse or smack your lips like you were blowing candles for a birthday or as if you had a plan to whistle.

4. Breathe slowly and exhale by exhaling through your lips with your purse or timer of four minutes.

After a morning's breathing technique or meditation, you can perform an easy stretching or range-of-motion practice while lying on your back.

Afternoon: Apply warmth to the site of pain over 6 to 10 minutes. If you experience high levels of pain, like 8-9 out of 10, it is possible to use an approach to a contrast bath that involves alternately cold and hot packs (2 minute hot and 2 minutes cold, for the total duration of 10 mins).

If you are lying on the ground and sitting down in a chair apply a light or moderate pressure to the area that is painful by using objects including an inflatable roller, rolled up towel, roll of paper towels or the rolling pin employed for baking.

Later in the evening, continue massaging the area of pain using various levels of pressure by using your hands or an instrument for massage. It is important to apply the appropriate quantity of pressure that's suitable for your body and isn't cause additional pain or discoloration of your skin. Also, you can incorporate other massage techniques including gentle lifting, pinching and moving the skin as much as you can.

Chapter 5: Learn About Other Types Of Pain

If you are trying to determine the cause of pain, understanding the different types of pain helps you to understand the causes for your body. You can then look into options to relieve pain and develop the ideal strategy. Furthermore, you'll be better able to describe what kind of pain that you're experiencing.

It's possible to have multiple types of pain-related symptom at the same moment. In this chapter, we will look at the four most common kinds of pain which a lot of sufferers experience. They are:

1. Pain that is referred

2. Pain that is not atypical

3. Pain from Neuropathic

4. Pain in the radicular region

The types of pain that aren't as prevalent include the visceral area or complicated regional painful syndrome (CRPS) that are covered in this chapter.

What is Referred Pain?

Referred pain happens where you experience pain on one part of your body, but the problem is caused by an entirely different source. This could be an indication of a severe or mild problem that you didn't initially consider.

It's not easy to identify referred pain however, being aware that referred pain is present could be life-saving. There are a few instances below to help you understand the concept of the concept of referred pain.

Anyone complaining of jaw pain the teeth or shoulder may possibly be suffering from an attack on the heart due to unblockage of the valves in the heart.

A pain in the neck could be caused by a range of things that originate from the lung, diaphragm, as well as the gallbladder and liver.

One less serious example of pain referred to is experiencing a brain freeze following eating ice cream that is cold. While the cold (ice cream) can be found in your mouth freezing sensation can be felt throughout your head.

The underlying cause of pain may be difficult to determine regardless of whether you attempt to imagine yourself as the therapy professional. Many therapists and doctors It's similar to putting together the jigsaw in a puzzle. We employ a variety of methods identify the root of the problem.

The chart below provides an example of pain points which could be caused through other parts within your body.

A region where pain is sensationally felt

The exact location where pain could originate

Shoulder

Liver, spleen, diaphragm

Back

Pancreas, kidney, stomach

Abdomen

Appendix, colon, Ovaries

Jaw

Heart

What is Nocieptive Pain?

Nociceptive pain can be felt in the event of an injury and the body's tissue has been damaged physically in any way. When you are injured and fall, twist your ankle, break your finger when cooking or twist your toe the discomfort you experience is called nociceptive pain.

Nociceptive pain can begin as acute pain that usually recovers within under 12 weeks. However, more serious injuries may persist, and cause permanent, chronic discomfort.

Since you're experiencing tissue damage and pain, it typically referred to as tightness, soreness the sensation of throbbing and pain.

It can also be disruptive to your daily routine It is characterized by inflammation, swelling, and bruising. The pain that you experience isn't due to nerve damage contrary to neuropathic pain.

What is Neuropathic Pain?

The treatment of neuropathic pain by certain practitioners and doctors is thought as a chronic illness that is a chronic condition. In order to better comprehend the effects of neuropathic pain on people, think of the following:

* Multiple cords of cable joined to a single cable box

They provide function to various rooms in your house.

Different cable cords get their signals from one box, allowing them to work correctly

A damaged one of the cables or a damaged cable box could affect the entire function

Pain from neuropathic causes in similar fashion. If there's injury or weakness within the nervous system, it is a sign of discomfort. It is comprised by the spinal cord, brain as well as peripheral nerves. The nerve fibers that are damaged in the nervous system transmit improper signals through the body. This can cause disturbance to your body's functions.

It is characterized by the presence of burning, tingling sensations of numbness or pins and needles as well as extreme cold or hot sensations. Other examples of neuropathy include:

* Neuropathy discomfort (tingling or sharpness on the feet and hands See chapter 4 for further details about neuropathy)

* Sciatic discomfort (tingling and burning sensations in the leg and back)

*Trigeminal nerve discomfort (facial burning, tingling hypersensation)

* Shingles, or any other infection that causes discomfort (tingling and numbness across the body)

What is Radicular Pain?

Radicular pain is experienced due to the fact that the spinal nerve has been damaged, compressed, or damaged or inflamed. It can also result as a result of a pinched spinal nerve, or from an impingement at all vertebrae (cervical and thoracic).

The pain starts in your hips and back but it radiates down your leg. It can be painful to sit for long time, walking on small distances, or engaging with basic activities and exercises quite difficult.

Radicular pain is also referred to by the name of "radiculopathy or sciatica pain". The term sciatica is often used due to the sciatic nerve's roots and pain is felt within the lumbar region of vertebrae. The sciatic nerve is the most long and largest nerve within the human body. It stretches through the middle of your leg and down to the foot, which is in the back of your body.

When the sciatic nerve becomes injured, it will spread throughout the body. But, the lower back area is usually affected by sciatica and radicular discomfort.

The pain of radicular enlargement is debilitating and can cause muscle weakness and difficulties in walking and standing most likely because many suffering from radicular pain suffer from bones spurs, herniated discs and spinal stenosis. The symptoms of pain could be, however, they aren't limited to numbness and tingling. the sensation of pounding or radiating.

Visceral vs. Somatic Pain

Numerous nurses, doctors, and therapists categorize pain into two general types, which they call "somatic" or "visceral" pain. There are distinct distinctions between these two categories and both can be classified as acute, short-term or chronic long-term discomfort.

Somatic pain can be described as a form of nociceptive pain. visceral pain is recognized by referring pain, and we've discussed both of the types of pain in greater specific detail in the previous chapter.

What is Somatic Pain?

Somatic pain can be experienced as a result of normal injuries, which can be felt in the superficial or deep areas of the muscles and joints. The most common type of somatic pain is "localized", which means that you can pinpoint where the pain is emanating from, and isn't spreading to other areas within your body. This differs from the deep somatic pain as it depends on the severity of trauma, the pain may become "generalized" and felt more widely around the injury area.

Common examples of injuries that cause mild somatic pain could be an injury to your skin while cooking, or a cut from an ankle sprain from an unintentional tumble. These types of injuries are distinct from the ones which cause deep somatic pain. It is also a common occurrence that will take a longer time to recovery.

Somatic pain that is deep originates from injuries that are located in the joints, bones and muscles. A few common injuries that could result in deep somatic pain be a rotator-cuff tendon tear, inflammation or scratches on your bones or within the joints. Pain that is caused by a somatic injuries can quickly turn into chronic pain if it is not addressed properly.

The symptoms of pain differ between deep and superficial pain. For superficial somatic pain may be intense burning, pricking or burning. deeper somatic pain may feel dull and sore. Whatever the characteristics of pain they can all differ in the intensity of pain.

What is Visceral Pain?

In contrast to somatic pain present in tisssues and tisssues visceral pain comes from the inner organs as well as structures in the body. The way in which the pain is are identical to the deep muscular pain that is dull and dull. It could also be accompanied by the sensation of pressure and cramping. It can also be characterized by squeezing, squeeze, turning and chewing. There may be visceral pain after a surgery. The most common reasons for visceral pain are:

Menstrual cramps

Problems with digestion, for example constipation

Tumors located in pelvis, back or abdominal area

Poor blood flow through the arteries

Organs are damaged by injuries like kidneys, gallstones and the liver

- appendicitis

- bowel blockages

Visceral pain can be linked with a different underlying issue that is well-known including IBS, cancer or heart problems. But, there are a few circumstances in which a person isn't aware of the cause of pain in the viscera. If that is the case it is often difficult to determine the exact location where the pain is occurring.

Contrary to the sensation of somatic pain that is superficial, visceral pain can radiate into various parts of the body. It is a part of "referred pain". It is the case it is when you think that it is originating in one part of your body, however the pain actually comes from a different part of your body.

Additionally, there can be related symptoms which can be accompanied by the visceral area, such as nausea and sweating as well as changes in heart rate and blood pressure.

Chronic pain in the viscera is believed to cause psychological harm on people. It could trigger major depression problems, anxiety, or sleep loss due to its complex nature. Your therapist may suggest that you seek medical assistance to treat chronic pain in the viscera.

Complex Regional Pain Syndrome (CRPS)

Complex Regional Pain Syndrome, often referred to CRPS is an rare diagnoses that therapists hate to be told about. If a person suffers from CRPS, that usually indicates that the symptoms are severe pain-producing and are confined on the arms, hands and legs, or feet. The symptoms of CRPS are however, not only these:

Hypersensitivity to the touch of your own touching

Mode to severe swelling

The skin's appearance appears smooth and soft

The skin's shade (ranging between blue and red or white)

The limitation of the active range of motion as well as joint stiffness in the body part affected

The skin temperature is felt either cold or warm

What is CRPS?

It can be triggered by something like a simple injured ankle or more severe than an attack on the heart. Medical scientists are still seeking to determine the cause and the reasons behind CRPS's development. The theory is that CRPS happens because of a malfunction within the peripheral or central nervous system (which comprises the spinal cord, brain and the extremities).

Additionally, research suggests that CRPS may be due to nerve dysfunction due to an injury in a body component. If therapists treat patients suffering from CRPS they will be diagnosed with "Type 1" or "Type 2".

Type 1 - Manifests when an illness or injury occurs that does not cause harm to nerves of the body area affected.

Type 2: Develops following the occurrence of a disease or injury and nerve damage occurs within the body part affected.

The pain from CRPS can be continuous and can get worse with the course of time. People who have CRPS report that their symptoms can feel as if they're experiencing pins and needles, or burning sensations that last throughout the day.

Together with occupational or physical therapy the majority of people suffering from CRPS are prescription medications from their physician to alleviate extreme pain.

Chapter 6: Preventing The Start Of Pain

Everyone has been told to keep a straight posture every day of our daily lives. Somebody in your circle might have told you "Don't to slouch. Make sure you sit up straight in your seat. Retract your shoulders, and straighten your head and neck." The truth is, we were advised this as it is painful to suffer long-term consequences of poor posture.

Develop the ability to think like a Therapist and follow plans before the pain starts. Joint protection, postural training as well as the conservation of energy are three techniques to stop pain from starting. The three strategies you can use include stretching your muscles and being logical about how you move during your day. These methods are simple to integrate into your daily routine. It will provide you with long-term, results that are positive.

What is Postural Training

Postural exercise helps reduce or alleviate persistent pain caused by disease and illness such as diabetes, arthritis, stroke, and more.

Postural training is the process of teaching your body how to stand, walk, stand and lay down in a way which will put the smallest amount of stress on your bones, muscles and joints.

What are the benefits of postural exercise? Since bad posture can result in physical and psychological negative results. Physically, poor posture may have a negative impact on confidence in yourself as well as convey to other people that you are lacking confidence and the strength. Physically, poor posture may result in curvature of your cervical spine, neck pain breathing issues, digestive disorders or sleep deprivation. It can also cause shoulder and hip painfulness.

A shoulder impingement that developed through poor posture could restrict the ability to reach to, hold or transport items. Take a look at the following postural methods for your daily routine to reduce the pain in your shoulder.

Start by standing up with your head in a straight line and shoulders pressed against the wall. The distance between your feet should be about one-quarter of an inch apart.

Move your arms upwards and downwards while sliding your body into the wall, for the minimum of 10 reps.

Other postural shoulder exercises for exercise involve the scapula that helps control the shoulder.

Begin: Stand up on your hands by your sides, looking ahead.

Moving: Bring your shoulders up and down to a minimum of 10 times.

Postural exercise could play an important role in the prevention of long-term neck pain as reducing tension. Do these neck movements.

Begin by sitting comfortably in a chair and place your hands placed on your lap or in the chairs' arms.

Moving: Move your head in a forward or backward direction and let yourself relax slowly while holding a 2 second stop.

The next step is to try an alternative neck motion.

Moving: Slowly move your head to the left and right, as if you're bringing your ear toward your shoulder as you allow yourself to hold for 2 seconds.

Instructing your pelvic muscles to work correctly, enhances posture overall. The center of your body is the pelvis. If you don't have stabilities in the core area the pelvis, discomfort is more likely to occur. We will go over methods to strengthen the core and pelvic muscles.

Check out these techniques for strengthening your postural muscles:

The first step is to lie in a position on your back without support. Allow you to take in a couple of deep breaths.

Move 1: Lean your knees towards the ceiling.

2. Place your feet flat on floor, with your hips spaced.

Third Movement: Place your legs straight across the floor with your arms at your side.

4. Then lift your pelvis up off the floor. Then, gently return it to the floor.

Perform this exercise as many times as you are comfortable with you. However, try to do 5-10 repetitions.

With time, and as you build up your tolerance levels, gradually increase the number of repetitions. Be sure to keep a the proper balance and form, such like the one shown in the image.

In training your abdominal and core muscles will help ease back pain and stabilize nearby muscles. Training your core and abdominal muscles can help improve posture in general.

This is where the "plank," can be executed in a variety of positions such as side either high or traditional using elbows, or on palms in the air. Here are the steps to perform the standard plank

Begin: Lay face-down on the floor.

First move: Place the weight of your upper body on bent elbows, pressing them against the floor

2. Press up by placing your feet on the floor while keeping the weight of your lower body onto your feet

Keep the posture for 15-30 seconds each time before you begin. After that, slowly raise the duration according to your comfort level.

The "high" plank differs from the standard elbow plank. When you do a high plank the arms are extended straight, and you place your hands laid flat on the floor (instead of putting weight onto your arms).

Your lower body stays in the same place that traditional planks are in; in both cases, your body remains set and aligned to straight up slope.

The angle of the "side" plank differs a little from "elbow and high" planks. Side planks help ensure that the spine is aligned. The following are steps to do the side plank:

Start by finding a comfy either right or left side in the ground.

Motion #1: Completely rest your body weight onto your elbow bent on the floor.

Second Movement: Place your body with upwards direction by lifting your hips and lifting your lower midsection off the ground.

Third Movement: Put your other hand onto your hip

Fourth Movement: Stay in the pose for a period of 15-30 seconds each time, gradual increasing your duration depending upon your individual tolerance.

Below are some other exercise routines for postural fitness focused on the glutes, core as well as hip muscles. These exercises prepare your body for sitting long periods of time. They also assist in improve the stability and strength of your the lower back muscles.

Begin by putting your back, comfortably lying on the floor, with your feet spaced slightly apart.

Move 1: With legs straight, elevate about an inch or so off the ground. Start abducting outward (abduct is the term used to describe pulling the leg away from your body) and then return into the opposite direction for 5-10 repetitions.

Second movement: Next move your leg upwards and then lower your leg to five to 10 reps. This is a more challenging move due to the fact that you're working against gravity.

3. Then you can reposition yourself lying on your back. Do leg lifts by lifting your leg up (towards towards the ceiling) in opposition to gravity for between 5 and 10 times.

Make rest breaks as needed then complete the three moves by using both feet.

Postural exercises can be completed either standing, sitting or lying down on the ground. As you work your body, you are moving through various positions which at first could cause discomfort. But, it is possible to notice some new signs of

tension, numbness and discomfort on specific body areas you weren't aware of.

Training in postural posture while sitting

These techniques offer effective exercise for your postural muscles while you sit. Sitting for too long in a chair (for instance, working in a computer every day) may cause muscular and back muscle pain.

A word of caution: Do not be in a seat for more than 30 to 45 minutes, without getting up up, moving or changing your posture.

Step 1: Design your own lumbar cushion by making a towel roll into the shape of a log.

Step 2: Put the towel on top of your buttocks, and then against your chair to strengthen the natural curve of the lumbar region.

Step 3: Put your feet in the chair and sit spine as straight as you can while your buttocks are touching the rear of the chair.

The next step is to practice training using exercises for lower back stretch in order to encourage good posture.

Motion 1: Sit at the edge of your chair and then put your feet flat on the floor and make sure your shoulders are aligned.

2. Slouch and lean forward while using your head, shoulders and neck (moving in a single unit).

Third Movement: Backwards stretch using your shoulders, your neck and head until your chest now sticks out.

Repeat the process for five to ten times.

Training in postural posture while standing

Here are some postural exercises to do when standing, which can help in relieving back pain. The exercises can are designed to stretch the back and arms in order to permit prolonged sitting as well as standing all day long.

First step: Grab the towel in a long way with your extended arms, while standing up.

Second Movement: Slowly strengthen your upper body, moving to the left, followed by on the left (apply for 3-5 seconds of rest).

Third Movement: Slowly move your body forward by tilting your body forward and then returning to your upright posture.

The next step is to practice postural methods in standing to help the lower body's balance and balance.

First step Start by standing with your feet about hip distance away. Flex your left knee, then grasp your left foot using the left hand.

First step: Stay in the posture for about 20-30 seconds while you place your opposite hand against a table, stool or even a wall, if required.

Second Movement: Repeat the procedure for the other side.

Training for postural stability while in the air

Here are some postural exercises that you can do on the floor using either a large towel or mat for help in relieving the stress and strain on your back and core muscles.

Begin by kneeling on the ground with your feet straight, hands placed flat to the ground. Before beginning the workout, be sure that you're feeling calm and not having breath that is too heavy.

Motion #1 Start by curving your back, after which straighten it 5-10 repetitions.

Then proceed to the next set of movements.

First step: Keep your right hand, while keeping your left foot, straight and in line with the floor Hold for 5 seconds.

Second movement: Return to the full kneeling position using both hands and knees placed on the floor.

3. Reverse your position by lifting your right hand and left foot off the floor directly out, in a straight line to the floor. keep them for five seconds.

What is Energy Conservation?

The term "energy conservation" refers to the practice of performing exercises and body routine activities during the day to reduce discomfort, joint and bone tension, muscle tear and fatigue.

Through implementing strategies and methods designed to conserve energy and energy conservation, you can increase your energy throughout the day. You will also reduce anxiety, stress and frustration.

Conservation of energy depends on planning (be sure to make plans for the future) and organisation. In particular, learning the right breathing methods to calm your mind will be beneficial when you discover you breathless at some point in the near future. Remember these tips while trying to reduce your energy consumption:

* Take care to balance rest and physical exercise in a balanced manner (too excessive of either one is not a good thing).

Do the work with a slower pace and make sure to take regular rest breaks.

Make sure you are using appropriate body mechanics in any physical activity, which includes at-home and workplace tasks.

Reduce the amount of lifting large objects by having them in an area that is easily accessible so that they don't cause strain.

• Only participate in the necessary physically beneficial activities.

If you have a typical 9-to-5 work schedule look into work-simplification techniques to save energy. This includes:

• Sit while working (instead of sitting) every time you are able.

• Delegate physical responsibility on to other people if you can.

* Only complete jobs that are essential to your work.

Utilize equipment whenever it is possible, making adjustments to the machine in order to reduce the amount of reach or exerting pressure you have to do in order when you are performing your job.

Make sure that you do not have to endure too much heat as extreme temperatures could rob you of your energy levels, and cause people feel tired or slow.

What is Joint Protection?

Joint protection can be a method to alleviate pain using an individual approach to managing your pain. It aids in preserving energy as well as improve joint performance. This approach to joint health is to apply it all day long. It is required to practice how to use the correct body mechanics and methods to conserve energy.

The most effective way of providing an effective method for joint safety is to get straight into it and offer you options to get involved in the process.

1. When you are able, utilize aidive equipment such as elevated seat for the toilet or shower benches, as well as hand-held reachers, and other equipment for cleaning.

2. If you cook, set up appliances like blenders to use on countertop in the kitchen (not

above the kitchen counters). Make sure you have aids like the jar openers in reach.

3. Make sure you have the strongest muscles and joints when lifting something.

4. Do the lifting near your body with your quads, legs or knees, not your back.

5. Utilize an unwheeled transporter.

6. Use both hands to carry items while pointing your palms upwards.

7. Make use of the lightest-weight items that you can.

8. You should sit whenever it is possible to ease the pressure on your hip joint and knee.

Chapter 7: What Exactly Is Peripheral Neuropathy (Pn)?

The peripheral neuropathy may result in your extremities becoming weaker as well as hurt. They can also become completely numb (typically around the feet and hands).

The brain and the spinal cord are able to communicate with other parts of your body through peripheral nerves. If those nerves get destroyed the messages they transmit are tampered by, affecting the way your body reacts to heat, pain and various other triggers.

Nerve damage in peripheral nerves is often the cause. Several reasons could lead to this injury:

The alcoholism and diabetes as well as infection

The adverse effects associated with peripheral neuropathy may strike abruptly or over time. There are many treatments that can be found dependent on the condition's root causes. A lot of natural and conventional solutions aim to ease the signs of pain.

Peripheral neuropathy symptoms

The symptoms of peripheral neuropathy vary based on the nature of the affected nerves. The three types comprise sensory nerves and autonomic nerves. Through relaying the instructions of your brain to muscles, your motor nerves help you to control your emotions.

If the motor nerves in your body have been damaged, you may suffer from these symptoms:

Are you having difficulty getting your legs or arms moving due to muscular atrophy or degeneration

Muscle spasms and uncontrolled twitching

The Sense Organs

Sensory nerves that send messages to your brain via diverse body organs, trigger the senses. If you experience coldness or whenever you touch something sharp the sensory nerves utilized.

If peripheral neuropathy is affecting the sensory nerves in your body, one of the following could happen:

The sense of touch is diminished. sensitiveness or tingling sensations.

The inability to feel pain as temperatures shift from cold to hot.

Reflexes and coordination are deteriorating.

Automatically you are tense

They regulate a variety of non-voluntary or partially voluntary activities that include the pulse rate, blood pressure, bladder function and sweating.

If your autonomic nervous system is affected by peripheral neuropathy you could experience the following signs:

A lot of sweating, lots of nausea, difficulty managing bladder and bowel movements as well as dizziness during standing or transferring from a seated position. A rapid heartbeat that is irregular and trouble swallowing

The kind of treatment you choose is dependent on the underlying nature of the peripheral neuropathy. The most commonly used treatments are surgeries, physical therapy and injections to boost the pressure on nerves. Some therapies aim to relieve pain and discomfort, as do over-the-counter medications like Ibuprofen and aspirin.

Coping and Managing Neuropathy

What factors can affect PN patients with depression and anxiety? It's not always clear how serious the PN symptoms can be! The most reliable predictors are psychological factors, or what do you think about? Negative or positive emotions social influences (such like "Are you active? ") or. Are you supported? Each of these aspects can be modified!

When you think about what might be the outcome if you had not been diagnosed, pity for yourself, reminiscing about the good times or seeing your self as an "PN patient," the burden of this illness can't be diminished. The coping strategies you employ are not effective and could make neuropathy-related symptoms get worse.

Here are some effective ways to cope and self-care:

The management of peripheral neuropathy

Some of the suggestions below can assist you in managing peripheral neuropathy

1. The maintenance of good foot health is essential if you suffer from diabetes. Check your feet on a regular basis for cuts, calluses, or blisters. Shoes and socks that are tight can cause the discomfort and cause tingling. They can also result in sores that will not get better. Use loose, comfortable wool socks, and shoes with padding. Utilize a semicircular hoop accessible in stores selling medical

supplies, for keeping bed sheets away from delicate or warm feet.

2. Stop smoking cigarettes; smoking may cause circulation problems, increasing the chance of having foot issues and even an amputation.

Get your nutrition in check; a balanced diet is essential in the case of chronic illness or you are at the highest risk of developing neuropathy. The diet you choose should consist of in fruit, vegetables Whole grains, whole grain, lower-fat dairy products, and meat foods. Drink alcohol only in moderation.

3. Massage You can give yourself an arm and foot massage or request a companion to help you. Massage can stimulate the nervous system, boosts circulation and can reduce discomfort temporarily.

4. Beware of pressure that is too intense; try not bent knees, or depending too heavily upon your elbows. It could cause injuries to the nerves.

Techniques for Peripheral Neuropathy Adaptation

Chronic or permanent pain can create daily difficulties. If you implement one or more of these strategies and techniques, you may be able to cope with the following issues:

Decide which chores, such as taking care of your bills or going through your grocery shopping, have to be done on a certain date and what tasks can be put off until later. Keep moving however, be careful not to overdo it.

Acknowledge and accept the negative effects of the situation in the present and continue to adopt an optimistic approach in order to discover what works for you.

Look for the positive aspects of this disorder. You consider it all bad. This could encourage you to keep a healthy routine, develop empathy more, or live a healthier way of life.

There's a tendency to go out on your own when experiencing a lot of discomfort, so you should take a break immediately. But, it's not difficult and helps you focus on your pain. Make a date with a person or watch a film or go for a walk.

Be active and create your exercise routine that is working to help you maintain your the highest level of fitness. It gives you an activity that you are able to manage, and offers a variety of effects on your mental as well as mental health.

Accept and seek help. seeking or taking help in times of need isn't a sign of vulnerability. As well as asking for assistance from your family members and friends Consider getting involved in a group of support to help those suffering from chronic suffering. While they may not be suitable for all people, support groups may help you learn ways to cope or treatment options that worked for some. Also, you'll get to meet others who know your situation. For information on a support organization that is in your local area, you can speak to your physician, a nurse, or even the nearby health agency.

Be prepared for difficult situations Being aware of what is required ahead of time will assist you in coping if something especially unpleasant, like the possibility of moving house or starting an opportunity to work, is expected to take place within your daily life.

Consult a counselor or therapist. The side symptoms of peripheral neuropathy may be depression, impotence as well as sleeplessness. If you suffer from one of these symptoms, it may be beneficial to talk with a counselor or psychotherapist along with your physician regarding your medical. Certain treatments can be beneficial.

Chapter 8: Sleeping Techniques For Neuropathy

As it helps to keep our bodies and minds working optimally and assists us in avoiding serious health issues, sleeping is a vital element of our daily lives. Every aspect of our mood like stress, mood, and even anxiety levels are impacted. Neuropathy often is a result of sleeping problems or insomnia. Patients who suffer from constant pain are often vocal about this problem.

More than 70% of sufferers, which includes those suffering from PN or back pain arthritis, and headaches as well as Fibromyalgia, have trouble sleeping, as per The Journal of Pain Medicine.

It is possible that pain will hinder you from sleeping because of a specific reason. Stress, anxiety, depression as well as the taking of drugs that disrupt sleep such as codeine make up the list of signs.

A majority of experts suggest 7 to 9 hours of sleep each every night, regardless of size or age. For those who are suffering from chronic pain, you might think that it is not possible, however there are things you could take to help improve the quality of your sleep. This can make you better and less nervous. Consult your physician to determine if there are any treatment options which can help reduce your sleep disturbed at first. In addition, it is important to consult with your physician to ensure that your medications may be the cause problems with your sleep.

There are many options you can try on your own to enhance your sleeping habits, besides using a medication. There are several methods to consider for you to go to sleep faster or sleep longer sleep, remain asleep and eventually, help you remain fit and healthy.

Here are some suggestions to assist you in sleeping better

Do not drink as much caffeine, particularly in the after-hours.

Quit smoking.

Reduce or eliminate alcohol consumption.

Ideally, limit nap times to not exceed one hour.

Beware of spending too long at night because prolonged inactivity during the night can result in a more shallow sleeping.

Keep a consistent daily program that incorporates the same sleep time and wake-up times.

Make sure you keep a consistent exercise routine ensure you train before you go to bed.

Be sure that the bed you sleep on is warm and comfortable. There should plenty of room for you to move and spread out comfortably. Test different mattress hardness options, egg-crate or foam toppers, as well as more comfortable pillows.

Make sure you have a cool and comfortable environment. the temperature of your room influences how much you rest. Most people who sleep in a space with good airflow and temperatures that is around 65 degrees F (18deg C) creates the most comfortable sleep environment. Insecure sleeping habits could be caused by your bedrooms.

Most people utilize computers as well as televisions to wind down after a hard day. So, they should be turned off. Alongside the fact that lighting can hinder the production of melatonin in humans, televisions is a great way to stimulate the mind, rather than relax it.

You should stop observing the clock and set your alarm clock to ensure it's not in front of you.

To allow you to note down your ideas that could cause you to be up all late at night, before putting them down, have an eraser and notebook close to the nightstand.

As the body needs the time to cool off before sleeping, you should avoid the use of a hot bath or shower prior to going to falling asleep.

Choose activities that relax you, for example, listening to relaxing songs or reading an audiobook.

Try to imagine a tranquil, serene setting. Relax your eyes, and attempt to imagine a calm and peaceful scene or activity. Think about how serene this scene or event can make you feel.

Some patients find the use of a cushion between their legs which stops the knees from touching one another can provide a sense of comfort. As long as you keep your leg from causing your spine to misalign in the evening, a cushion put between your legs will reduce tension on your hips and lower back. It can take between three and four weeks of following these methods before you can notice changes in your sleep.

Chapter 9: Maintaining A Healthful Lifestyle

Physically fit as well as being mentally and emotionally sound is a must for being healthy. A healthy lifestyle should be element of your life. Healthy living can aid to prevent the development of chronic diseases and debilitating ailments. What you think of yourself as well as how take care of your mental and physical health determines your degree of self-esteem as well as self-image. Maintaining your health is vital to living an appropriate lifestyle.

The Impact Of Attitude

Positive outlooks can increase your confidence, increase the strength of your soul, encourage others and help you gain the strength to conquer obstacles. A minor shift in perspective can make a big difference.

Healthier relationships, healthier as well as greater achievement is strongly linked to being optimistic. Based on certain research the personality traits of optimism and pessimism can affect various aspects of your health and wellbeing. A positive attitude to manages stress is essential to its efficacy. An optimistic approach will boost the energy of your body, increase your own strength, motivate people around you, and provide the determination to conquer obstacles. The research shows that thinking positive will prolong your lifespan, ease the burden of despair, improve the physical and mental health of your and assist you in dealing in the face of stress and hardship more efficiently. Stress management that is effective also offers several health benefits.

Here are a few ways of creating a positive attitude:

Self-talk: The initial step towards positive thinking involves self-talk. Self-talk refers to an ongoing, daily uninterrupted thought stream that flows through your mind. It is possible to come up with some positive or negative thing that you think of. The use of logic and reason for some of the statements you tell yourself. The false assumptions you make due to a lack of comprehension could result in different self-talk.

Make sure you surround yourself with positive people. Make time for people who inspire, are happy and energetic. Keep in mind that if one approaches someone who's drowning in the water too much, he or might drag you alongside the person. Opt to be a positive individual rather than a negative one. Make sure you're happy in your own skin. If you're not looking to surround yourself with negative people Why do you believe that other people would? You can take back control of your mind.

Be aware of your negative thoughts:

For this purpose to achieve this, these strategies may be used:

Try viewing it as half full instead of half empty.

Try to get the most effective result.

Keep a middle-ground approach Don't get amazing or terrible views regarding all things. This means that it is possible to reduce the highs and lows.

Be aware of negative thoughts and becoming aware of them whenever they come up. This way it is possible to change your behaviour.

Unfortunately, there are some who have the worst attitude towards them. Try to be kind to yourself. The truth will begin to sink in when you constantly critique yourself. The negative thoughts can make you feel depressed in the long run. Maybe it's an ideal time to engage those who are supportive rather than critique.

Make realistic goals that are achievable There's no need to set unrealistic expectations, as provided you don't make a fuss of yourself for not meeting the goals. It will boost your confidence when you establish realistic goals and make a lot of singles, instead of playing for fences.

Think about the bigger picture: Success in your life is establishing goals and focusing efforts in the areas you want to focus on. It's important to not allow little incidents that occur each day cause you to be unhappy. You can move on once you have learned how to deal with or brush off any minor problems. The time has come to concentrate on the important aspects.

Make challenges opportunities Instead of letting the challenges take over your life, transform challenges into opportunities. (To stay away from falling over the wall, walk over or evade the wall.)

There are plenty of blessings to be thankful for Be grateful for them instead of neglecting them. People can accomplish this through expressing gratitude around the table at dinner writing a journal, or posting the most memorable event or activity every daily on Facebook. Be aware that not all the greatest things that you can have in your life are tangible. Make every opportunity to create your own unique life experience.

It's not clear why people who are positive enjoy these benefits. A theory suggests that an optimistic outlook can help to handle stressful circumstances better, which in turn reduces the detrimental impact of stress on the health of your body. In addition, studies suggest that people who are happy and cheerful are healthier, as they take more exercise, eat healthier as well as don't smoke and aren't drinking excessive alcohol.

Help on how to handle the strain of having peripheral neuropathy, while taking good care of your physical requirements daily.

Therapy and physical activity

A physical exercise routine can assist in retain strength, mobility and functioning regardless of primary cause for peripheral neuropathy (PN). In order to avoid severe changes, diabetics need to be vigilant about checking for blood sugar level. The physical therapy could aid patients suffering from diabetic neuropathy too.

A few of the goals of physical therapy are these:

Utilizing a passive range of motion in order to increase and preserve the range of motion Self-stretches and progressive stretching are just a few of the exercises.

Weightlifting, isometric exercises as well as working out using increasing resistance are just a few exercises that build muscle strength.

Through balance training, stabilization and fall prevention can be achieved.

The physical therapist may suggest braces or splints for aid in balance and posture.

Splints are frequently utilized as a treatment for mononeuropathies of compression, including carpal tunnel syndrome.

Chapter 10: Improving Sensory-Motor Skills

Instructing patients to be aware of toxic substances in the air or from industries

Practicing self-care methods

Informing the general public on patient health concerns (e.g. paying greater focus on the ground when walking, as slipping or falling can be dangerous to patients suffering from PN) instructing the patient to pay attention to issues that affect autonomic functioning (e.g. the ability to move around without a hitch so as to minimize an abrupt decrease in blood pressure, and the possibility of falling)

Exercising Aerobically

The heart rate, breathing rate and muscle contractions will all rise. The majority of people are advised to try to do a minimum of 30 minutes per day between 3 and 5 times each week. If you're not in the past, you can start by doing just 5 to 10 minutes each every day. Then, increase it throughout the week.

Also, you can break your daily exercises into smaller portions. Take a for instance, 10 minutes of exercise right after eating.

Here are a few instances of exercise that is aerobic:

Participate in a low-impact aerobics class or go for a walk (on an exercise bike or in the outdoors).

You can swim or exercise inside the pool or using a stationary bicycle.

Flexibility Education

Training for flexibility and maintenance can help keep joints flexible and lower your chance of getting injured while doing other physical activities. If you can stretch your muscles for five to 10 minutes Your body will begin to get warm and fit for aerobic exercises such as swimming or walking. Here are a few stretches that you can practice at home in order to increase the flexibility of your.

Make sure to consult your physician prior to beginning any workout program.

Increasing plantar fascia elasticity

When you are facing the door frame, you should place your foot as close to the frame as possible. While your heel is dangling forward and your feet pointing towards the sky, slowly lean toward the forward. For a longer stretch by bending your front knee toward your door's frame. Your heel cord and muscles of the sole of your feet are likely to be stretched. Perform 3 times of each leg to get a 15 second rest every each day.

while you are seated when seated, stretch your hamstrings

Lengthen one leg straight while pointing your foot upwards as you sit in front of an upright chair. While you bend the opposite knee, the foot should rest flat to the ground. As you slowly straighten your back, making sure your chest is directly above the straight leg until you feel the stretch at the rear side of your leg. Each leg should last fifteen to twenty minutes. Complete 3 repetitions for each leg, twice daily.

Extended Calf

The toe on one leg is to be pointed towards the back and extended in front of your back. Begin the process by using your opposite foot. Move forward, keeping your knees slightly bent while your back foot is firmly set on the ground. The back leg's calf area will appear stretched. On each leg, you should rest for 15-20 minutes. Do 3 repetitions of each leg three times daily.

Strengthening Exercises

The practice of doing exercises to build muscles' strength and resistance to injury. The way to recover the strength of your muscles by adhering to an workout regimen. Here are some exercises for strengthening you can try at the comfort of your own home.

Make sure to consult your physician prior to beginning any workout program.

Raising Countertop Calf

While at the counter Place two fingers' tips onto the counter. Move the heel of the foot over to the side and stand on your feet (as you work your muscles, change your heels, as illustrated in the image below). Then slowly lower yourself down to the ground, and then continue to do it. After you're on your feet, slowly reduce your weight. Never give up and relax. Repetition 10 to 15 daily at least twice for each leg. Perform 3 times of each leg to get a 15 second rest every two days.

Sofa Squat

Choose a comfortable chair that has armrests. Position your feet with a split stance with one leg in the middle of the chair, and one foot placed to the front and slightly towards the sides. Slowly shift your weight to the side until your legs support all of your body weight. Gradually raise your legs until they sit. Slowly lower yourself until your hips rest against the chair. In the next rep put your legs against the chair. Then lift yourself to the top. Do not rest between sets as well as "plop" in a chair. Between 15 and 10 times. daily for 2 repetitions two times. Each leg should last fifteen to twenty minutes. Do 3 repetitions of each leg, twice daily.

The back of the chair is extended

You should sit on the front of the chair with both feet directly on the ground. Then slowly lift the ankle up and toes in the highest position you can. Let them fall slowly. In order to make the exercise more difficult, keep the feet into a tight place. Two times daily 10 to 15 times at least three times per week.

Balance

If you experience indications of illness, such as joints that are painful, weak, or dizziness, keeping an appropriate balance is crucial. There is a chance that you can overcome stiffness or unsteadiness through practicing balance. In older individuals particularly it is the role of balance that plays an larger and greater function. The risk of falling is higher due to the fact that older muscles are less agile smaller and less sensitive when you have to stabilize your body.

Raising Countertop Calf

While at the counter At the counter, put the tips of your fingers across the countertop. Move the heel of your foot towards the opposite side, while sitting with your feet on the floor (as you work your muscles, you can change your heels, as illustrated in the image below). Then slowly lower yourself down to the floor and continue to do it. After you've landed on your feet, slowly reduce your weight. Do not give up, and lie down. Repetition the exercise ten to fifteen times during the course of the day. Repeat twice for each leg.

Extended Hip

If you are steady, perform your task while holding the chair or table using the one hand, the tip of one finger, and finally not holding anything. Keep your body straight and use tables or chairs to aid in balance. Lean one leg in a gentle manner towards the chest, without bent the legs or the waist. Keep the leg in this position for five to 10 minutes. Slowly lowering your leg is recommended. Continue with the next leg. Then, hold for five to ten minutes. Repeat the exercise twice daily at least once for each leg.

Increased Hip

If your body is stable, do the exercise while holding your table or chair with just the one hand, using the tip of one finger, and finally with no hold whatsoever. Establish the distance between 12 to 18 inches from your feet to table or the chair. When you are benting your hips, secure yourself to the chair or table. Take one leg and slowly lift it move it back. Keep your body in a position for 5-10 seconds. Continue with the second leg, progressively lower the previous. Do this for 5-10 minutes. Do 2 sets on each leg. Repeat twice daily.

lateral leg lift

If you're stable, do the exercise while holding your chair or table using the one hand, one fingerstip at the end, but without any other objects. Stand straight and set your feet in a space in front of a table or chair. Take a table or chair to the balance. Then slowly raise the leg about 6-12 inches towards the side. Do the same with the second leg as you gradually lower the previous. Make sure your back and knees are straight during exercise. Keep your hands on the floor for five to 10 minutes. Repeat this twice daily twice on each leg.

Nutrition

An enlightened diet is often the initial option to protect yourself from many ailments, like PN. Find out ways to reduce the effects of drugs as well as shop and maintain an appropriate food plan.

Chapter 11: Peripheral Neuropathy And Diet

An enlightened diet is often your first option to protect yourself from many ailments, which includes peripheral neuropathy. If you are looking to reduce the risk of peripheral neuropathy, you must take care to manage the medical issues that place your health at high risk. If you are diabetic that means you must control the blood sugar levels, or if you believe that you may have an alcohol dependence issue, talk with your physician about treatment options that are safe and efficient. No matter if you're suffering from an illness or not, you should eat an energizing diet filled with fruits, vegetables as well as whole grains and protein that is lean. Maintain a food journal to track the foods you consume and ensure that you are getting the daily minimum amount of nutrition to be healthy.

Note: Always consult your physician prior to beginning any supplement or diet regimen.

Dietary Principles for Nerve Health

If you suffer from a neurological illness, eating a diet high with particular nutrients can prove beneficial. Food choices will improve the way the nervous system works. Being healthy as well as reducing the chance of suffering from nerve related issues can be possible if you know what foods you should eat in order in order to strengthen the nervous system.

Lean protein and whole cereals, legumes, grains and vegetables are the basis of your daily diet.

Eat 5-10 portions of bright fruits and/or vegetables per daily (phytonutrients). Serving sizes of all fruit and vegetables equals to 1 cup.

One medium-sized fruit or vegetable for example, such as an apple or an orange.

Dry fruits 1 cup

A quarter cup juice

Beware of or avoid the consumption of alcohol.

The impact of toxicology on nerve tissues

Be aware of your intake of salt and aim to ensure that you consume 2300 mg a day.

Reduce the consumption of trans and saturated fatty acids by selecting lean meats and poultry as well with dairy that is low in fat and non-fat items.

Replace saturated and trans fats with mono- or polyunsaturated oils (found in nuts, fish as well as the oils of vegetables).

Select or cook foods and beverages that have little or the absence of added sugars or calorie sweeteners.

Inflammation-Reducing Food

The chronic low-level inflammation can be found deeply below the surface of the skin that it can't be observed or perceived. The immune system is in overdrive and damages healthy tissues can lead to long-term diseases. Use the following guidelines to minimize inflammation to the maximum extent possible:

Consume more omega-3 fatty acids:

Each day, eat 1 to 2 teaspoons flaxseed (grind the seeds to maximize effect)

Take fatty fish every two weeks that weighs up to 3-4 pounds. (include wild mackerel, halibut and salmon and tuna)

3 ounces of walnuts per every day

The antioxidants and fiber are:

Enhance the amount of antioxidants found in vegetables and fruits (at at least 5 a each day):

Eat foods that slowly allow nutrients to enter your bloodstream (fruits and vegetables nuts, beans, and seeds)

The Best Diet for Blood Sugar Control

Blood sugar levels that are elevated can affect a variety of chronic illnesses, such as peripheral neuropathy caused by diabetes. In order to help manage your diabetes, and to maintain the blood sugar levels that are at their highest,

Recognize Your Carbs!

foods that are rich in starch can include cereals, bread pasta, dried beans lentils, rice milk, juices of fruit, yogurt and various dairy products and sweets such as candies, cookies sweets, sodas that are regular, syrup and sugar.

Beans/fruits, whole grains and low-fat dairy items are examples of top-quality products.

Quantity: Record the carbs you consume, and look up the labels for the size of your portion and total carbs.

Technique of the Plate (half the plate with vegetables with a quarter cup of starch and one quarter of protein lean)

How to distribute portions of carbohydrate (3 smaller meals, 2-4 smaller snacks)

Taking Care of Treatment or Drug Side Effects

Life-threatening or long-term conditions often are prone to harm healthy cells too and can cause negative side effects from medications or treatments prescribed for treating the condition. Certain side effects may could cause eating disorders.

To reduce nausea, eat frequently and not feeling hungry in between meals, take 6-8 smaller meals consisting of simple foods.

Loss of weight that's unfavorable nutritious fats to your diet including avocado and olive oil, as well as nuts and seeds.

Constipation You should drink more water and fiber and eat more often.

If you suffer from diarrhea, you should avoid dairy products, and consume simple food items that are bland and low-fat.

How to Develop Peripheral Neuropathy Disease

Through Food is the Worse

The effects of alcohol, diabetes, trauma injury, vitamin deficiencies as well as other diseases can all cause PN. The treatment options are managing the underlying reasons, physical therapy medication, and changes to diet. To get the most effective outcomes, consult your physician.

Gluten consumption could worsen celiac symptoms or gluten sensitivities. The most common sources are anything made by mixing wheat, white cake flour, or baking powder. The products that advertise "gluten-free" should be sought for.

Due to the fact that refined grains are high in the glycemic index they have a significant impact on the levels of blood sugar. Controlling the levels of your blood sugar is your best protection against the development of diabetic neuropathy. To reduce the effects on your diet's glycemic index swap refined grains in favor of whole grains.

Although they can enhance the flavor of food, sugars added to drinks are deficient in nutrition. Insufficient nutrition may cause neuropathy-related signs. Make sure you are eating healthy foods such as fruits as well as vegetables, along with whole grains.

Saturated fats, commonly found in fat-rich meats and dairy products, could create inflammation and raise the likelihood of getting Type 2 diabetes. To maintain a healthy lifestyle the consumption of lean proteins should be used instead of fat-based ones and healthy fats should be consumed with moderation.

Food and Shopping - Be aware of the amount of liquid and food you consume in addition to your level of activity.

Shopping guides will allow you to plan your meals and help you make the right choices in the store. Create a list of all the items you'll need and adhere to it in order in order to stop impulse spending.

Supplements

The very first vitamin group which could prove beneficial to patients suffering from peripheral neuropathy are those belonging to that of the B vitamins. The B vitamin imbalance, specifically B-12 deficiencies, are often the reason for PN. Deficiency in B-12 can result in permanent nerve damage if not dealt with immediately. Food sources that provide the best source of B-12 include meat and fish, eggs as well as low-fat dairy products refined cereals, as well as meals made of dairy that are low in fat. For those who strictly eat vegetarians Fortified cereals can be an excellent source of vitamin B12. However, you might also wish consult with your physician concerning supplements to B-12.

It's not common to have vitamin E deficient, unless indigestive malnutrition or intestinal microbial absorption but vitamin E can be beneficial to treat PN.

Caregiver

We all at the time of our lives have to be or need to become an caregiver. What are you able to do to locate the right caretaker for you or your family member who suffers from an illness or disability that is chronic as well as what you can take to reduce the risk of "burnout" if you are taking care of someone else?

Chapter 12: Trying To Find A Caregiver

As independent as you are able to. But, asking for help could be useful if have difficulty with everyday chores. Remember these important tips before you hire the services of a caregiver

Consider whether you'll depend on relatives or an employee. Check the qualifications of candidates like their driver's license and insurance for liability, prior to making a decision to hire the person.

Find a partner whom you can trust and who is comfortable with. Are they able to communicate effectively? Are language barriers present? Are you awed by them?

Join as to form a tag group. When a lot of care is required for a caregiver, more than one could be required. If you are in a situation of crisis, having an emergency backup plan is beneficial.

Set out your expectations clearly. Does your caretaker cook? Clean? do tasks? If you've hired someone to do so, be sure you've made a note of the tasks they will be performing and stay up contact at a professional level.

Finding a Caregiver

A lot of caregivers, particularly relatives, experience feelings of desperation, heightened anxiety, and a general feeling that they are overwhelmed in caring for someone that is chronically sick or has disabilities. Here are some suggestions that can help reduce the mental and physical strain that comes with caring for a patient. There is numerous options and services to assist you in caring for the loved ones.

Join a support group for caregivers and don't lose your wit. If you are unsure of the kind assistance you need Be positive. Increase your self-efficacy and the conviction that you can manage and implement steps to address specific issues.

Contact your family or group for advice.

The setting of priorities can help you to manage your work load.

The importance of self-care

Be sure to consume a healthy diet, do regular exercising, and make sure you get plenty of rest. It is important to be happy with the work you manage to complete successfully. Bring joy to your daily life. Find something that you love to do everyday, whether that's gardening, watching films, or enjoying music

.

Start a journal

The writing process allows you to communicate your feelings and get a an understanding.

Find a way to relax (it is a process that requires time and time and practice).

Being a competent patient or caregiver demands that you prioritize your own needs. If you're the patient the caregiver knows how to offer you the greatest freedom. If you're the caregiver, you'll be a compassionate and nurturing support to the patient, while paying attention to your personal needs.

Natural remedies for peripheral neuropathy symptoms

The symptoms of peripheral neuropathy can be controlled organically by various methods:

1. Vitamin

Deficiencies in vitamin levels can cause peripheral neuropathy. B vitamins are essential to build powerful nerves. In the event of a deficiency, it could severely damage the nerves.

Vitamin B can be present in foods but your doctor might also advise using an supplement. To avoid toxicity or aggravation of symptoms, you must follow the dose guidelines.

Vitamin D is also able in preventing neural pain. The skin produces vitamin D upon exposure to the sun's rays. Insufficient levels can cause irritation in patients suffering from neuropathy. A supplementation program can ease neuropathy-related symptoms.

2. Chili pepper

Cayenne peppers contain the same chemical compound called capsaicin also present in all hot peppers. Capsaicin is a component of cosmetic creams because of its capability to reduce discomfort. It decreases the intensity of the signals that the body sends out.

Cayenne pepper is consumed as well as capsaicin pills that can be used to alleviate the pain of neuropathy.

Capsaicin-based ointments for topical use can be applied to the body. While it might be uncomfortable initially, usage will eventually reduce neurological symptoms.

Make sure you review the treatment program with your physician prior to beginning to ensure that you do not suffer negative consequences.

3. Stop smoking.

Smoking can affect blood circulation. Small blood vessels take in lower levels of oxygen. If the blood circulation in your body isn't working properly, then the peripheral neuropathy could worsen the pain and numbness it already feels. It is possible to see a decrease in the symptoms when you quit smoking. Consider this as an incentive to get better.

4. The steamy tub

Relaxing warm baths can be beneficial in reducing symptoms of neuropathy. Warm water boosts the flow of blood through the body. This decreases the pain that is caused through nerve numbness.

If peripheral neuropathy is affecting the sensory nerves in your body and you're less tolerant to temperature, take care not to get the bath too hot.

5. Exercise

Regular exercise is beneficial to overall health, and aid you with reducing discomfort.

Exercise can lessen the risk of nerve injury by decreasing glucose levels. Furthermore, exercising decreases stress and boosts the flow of blood into your legs and arms. All of these factors work to reduce pain and discomfort.

5. Plants that smell

Essential oils such as Roman camomile and lavender help improve the flow of blood throughout the body. They also possess anti-inflammatory and alleviating properties to assist in the healing process.

1 one ounce of carrier oil for example olive oil must include a couple of drops of essential oils. The application of these oils diluted on the area affected may assist in relieving the symptoms associated with peripheral neuropathy.

7. Self-reflection

Methods of meditation can aid sufferers of neuropathy manage their symptoms of pain. They can assist you in coping more effectively with stress, increase the way you deal with stress and reduce the severity of discomfort. Mind-body strategies are an effective non-invasive treatment that can provide the user with greater control over the situation.

8. Acupuncture

It promotes the healing process by activating the body's tension points. In this way the nervous system stimulates the release of chemical substances which can alter the way painful stimuli are perceived, or how much pain-inducing stimuli are accepted. Acupuncture can help the body's energy equilibrium, which can impact your mental well-being.

When compared to treatments the prevention method is better. A healthy blood sugar level can help prevent your neuropathy from getting worse. If drinking alcohol has contributed to the neuropathy you suffer from, stop drinking immediately to stop it from deteriorating.

Pain from peripheral neuropathy is successfully treated using home remedies. Consult your physician before starting a new treatment program to ensure your security. If you notice your symptoms beginning changing after utilizing herbal remedies or become worse, seek out a physician promptly.

Here are some healthy ways of living that will help you to be a well-balanced and healthy individual:

Maintain A Regular Exercise Routine.

There's no need for you to exert yourself to give everything in the gym, however it is still important to stay active as long as you are able to. Keep active through simple floor exercises or walking, swimming and doing some chores around your home. Pay attention to the signals your body sends.

Continue to maintain the exercise program you have been following. You should give yourself three or five times every week to workout for at least 20 to thirty minutes. Create a plan and be certain you exercise daily.

Pay Attention To Your Diet.

There's no need to be a slave to giving the best effort during your workout in the gym, however it is still important to stay going as hard as you are able to. It is possible to stay fit through simple floor exercises or walking, swimming and even doing household chores around your home. Be aware of your body's signals.

It is essential to keep up the routine of exercise. Make sure you give yourself three or five times each week to work out for a minimum of twenty-to thirty minutes. Set a timetable and make certain you exercise daily.

In order to avoid the stress of life's demands, you should indulge in the things you love to do and make time to enjoy something that you love.

Connect with people who inspire you

In order to be in a healthful physical and mental state You must be at peace and in a good energy state. There are many issues that are avoidable. However, it is beneficial to keep an optimistic attitude when you face the difficulties. Make time for people that will inspire you as well as others who may occasionally give some constructive feedback so you can get better.

Develop a routine to look at the positive side of everything. Even in the most dire of scenarios it is possible to find something positive to the scenario, something that is constructive and positive. Think about these concepts for more.

Healthy living isn't hard or arduous to maintain. It is possible to build a balanced persona by continuing to do the way you're going and utilizing these tips to stay fit.

Chapter 13: Medical Condition

What follows is my conclusion from the nerve conduction test as well as an electro-physiological test conducted by a physician at the University of Miami and that took about an hour. The outcome was:

1. Electroneurophysiological evidence was found of a primarily small fiber sensor neuropathy that affects the sympathetic part over the parasympathetic component leading to significant loss of the axon.

2. The right median nerve is affected in the wrist (carpal tunnel) which causes small sensory axon degeneration.

3. The right ulnar nerve is affected at the elbow that results in a mild loss of sensory axon.

Diagnosis: small fiber neuropathy.

It is a medical term and explained to the patient it is a sign that autonomic nerves were affected. tiny fibers, and lost axon, which means there was no connection connecting my nerve system to brain, and peripheral neuropathy as well. The symptoms I experienced are, as you can see are varied, apart from the typical pains associated with nerve pain and burning sensations in my feet and hands. My blood pressure fluctuated and my heartbeat fluctuated My digestive system did not transmit the message to my brain about what I was eating. This means that it didn't properly digest food, the gallbladder was functioning below norms it didn't sweat and the moment I was exposed to a extreme temperatures, I felt like I was in an oven. In the frigid temperatures, I could feel my skin burning the fingers turned red because the blood vessels that expand or contract to regulate your body's temperature failed to do so as they did not receive the message from the brain. Sometimes I experienced a loss of body temperature, so I needed to soak in warm water and heat my body to recover heat and I experienced sensitivity to the dark and occasionally noticed that my vision was blurry at night. I couldn't rest well as simply going to bed brought the pain to my entire body. My mind also became obscured. I would perform three tasks at the simultaneously, but I couldn't do any of them, at times, I was afraid that I would feel faint it was like my soul had fled the body. no bone inside my body that wasn't in pain or have a muscle or legs that were shaking. most concerning for me was the burning sensation that arose in my entire body. It was enjoyable, and their telling you there is no cure is a bit more gruelling and on the other side what prescribed is medications that harm the nervous system. I have never taken them and preferred living with pain as my objective was to re-establish my nervous system, and regain my health. At the very least I would like to test it. It comes to a point when you become accustomed to having suffering. Some days were that were better than others, however my faith and belief in recovery were higher which I was able to achieve. Nowadays, the majority of those signs are gone. I am able to walk and be active, and that it has improved by 90% and I'm hopeful of getting better because I'm planning continue to study. There's always the possibility of a bright future, so don't let it go!

In the future, I'll describe details of each of the supplements I took in order to help restore the vitality of my nervous system, and the ones that are most efficient. Every one of you can be able to make your own decision and determine if you'd like to test them out or not. We won't refer to a particular brand as I don't want people to believe that I'm promoting the product Keep in mind two factors, one thing is that the product is 100 percent organic and is a product that has the USDA certification, as some claim to be organic but aren't. Another thing to consider is looking at the list of ingredients Many products advertise that they are "organic apple powder" and in the table of ingredients, you will see additional herbs. The same goes for chemicals or supplements that are well-studied will reveal that the most that you're consuming is applesauce, and in the absence of being a healing agent, it can harm you. Check that the bottle is only containing all of the ingredients you're looking for. Be conscientious and faithful to the supplement, as you need to use the product daily for a few months for complete healing as your body needs time to heal. Do you realize that the nerve system is regenerated every eight months? The myelin that is lost within nerves isn't able to recover over the course of a day. That is why it takes a long some time. They are all natural except one I'll define clearly, to me, it's one of the main. You will begin seeing improvements in the second week, regardless of which type of neuropathy are suffering from, the process is exactly in the same way.

PRODUCT DETAILS

EMBLICA OFICINALIS. That's the scientific term and one to look through in the ingredients table. It is the only one that includes 100% emblicaofficinalis.

It's also called AMLA, AMALAKI, INDIAN GOSEBERRY

IT IS A PLANT THAT GROWS IN THE FORESTS OF INDIA AND PRODUCES FRUITS OF A VERY RICH YELLOW GREEN COLOR IN JUICES FULL OF HEALTH BENEFITS. ACCORDING TO THE INDIAN TRADITION, THE AMLA WAS THE FIRST TREE OF THE UNIVERSE AND HAS BEEN USED FOR THOUSANDS OF YEARS FOR THE TREATMENT OF DIFFERENT DISEASES THANKS TO THE ACTIVE PRINCIPLES THAT IT CONTAINS, LIKE VITAMIN C, BIOFLAVONOIDS, SAPONINS AND TANNINS, UNTIL THE POINT OF BEING CONSIDERED BY INDIAN POPULAR MEDICINE AS "THE TREE OF LIFE". IT HAS BEEN USED BY AYURVEDIC MEDICINE FOR THOUSANDS OF YEARS TO REJUVENATE THE BODY AND STRENGTHEN THE IMMUNOLOGICAL SYSTEM.

MANY RESEARCH ON AMLA AND CLINICAL STUDIES AND TRIALS ON HUMANS HAVE BEEN AFFECTED SPECTACULAR HEALTH BENEFITS.

The effectiveness of the extract amla for treating arthritis, hay fever osteoporosis, and joint pain has been proved.

DIABETIS; assists in regulating the metabolic process of carbohydrates, and boosts the uptake of glucose by cells. This helps to reduce the sugar levels in blood. This is helpful for patients who suffer from diabetes 2 because it regulates the hormone insulin.

Patients with diabetes should consult their doctor prior to using it since it may affect the medication prescribed in that it can block the effects of specific medications.

Amalaki may lower blood pressure therefore its use isn't advised for those with lower blood pressure. In this instance I have lower blood pressure and it did not affect the blood pressure of my patients.

The amla may also be indicated in the following situations:

Anti aging

General weakness Fatigue, general weakness

Tissue deficiency

Protector of the liver (weakness in the liver or the spleen)

Hepatitis

Hemorrhages

Hemorrhoids

Anemia

Gout

Vertigo

Gastritis

Osteoporosis

Constipation

Premature gray hair

States with fever

Mental disorders

Palpitations

While there aren't any warnings or contraindications to Amla it is a fruit to be handled with care. There is a risk of stomach irritation and irritation to the digestive tract and the risk of a decrease of blood pressure. My experience was that I did not feel any of these issues however any excess of it is harmful. For me, it was a great help greatly with the signs of neuropathy. But my primary reason for liking it was that it sucked away the burning sensation throughout my body in general, and as a result, I felt happy.

I drank it daily throughout the morning. I never consumed before sleep because the large amount of vitamin C could damage teeth enamel. In addition the ability to consume it anytime of your day, if it suits your needs. Don't mix it with yogurt or milk. I would recommend powder that is made from organic ingredients and mixing it with juice. However, the flavour isn't the most pleasant however the most effective way I could find to lessen its taste was to mix it with mixed juices made from strawberries, blueberries, blackberries and raspberries. Also, I suggest mixing it with blender since amalaki powder isn't diluted quite easily.

1/2 cup mixed fruit (mentioned in the previous paragraph)

One cup of water

1 teaspoon powder of amalaki

I have added sugar since I cannot stand drinking juice with no sweets, I am aware that some would think that this isn't nutritious and there's all that debate however I won't claim to be a person who is healthy and eats a balanced diet, in reality, I'm not a diabetic The choice now is yours to choose for each of you. Some are able to drink the juice without adding sugar some prefer to sweeten the drink. You can choose healthy options including stevia, organic honey, agave (that is my preferred should I have to pick) and honey. You can choose what you prefer. Limit yourself to one teaspoon of amalaki powder daily okay?

I used it for about one month, and after that I stopped taking again until I started feeling those symptoms once more. It is advisable to take it off for a time and then begin the next cycle after about a month. This will depend on your body's tolerance to it. After all, it is a fruit. However, there are some fruits that do not be a hit with all people equally.

HERICIUM ERINACEUS The scientific name. Check the list of ingredients because often they combine it with vitamin D and other ingredients. Be aware of this because it's the one that's most vital and is the one that aids in the regeneration of your nervous system.

It's also known as MELENA DE LEON The name is the LION'S MUSHROOM, YAMABUSHITAKE.

Lion's Mane is an ancient Chinese medicinal fungus widely identified as a supplement with numerous advantages. The neuroprotective properties that it has proven and its ability to boost the creation of nerve growth factor (NGF) makes the Lion's Mane an extremely sought-after and effective natural nootropics. Recent research suggests the fact that Lion's Mane extract improves nerve growth factor (NGF) production. It is an amino acid is found in the brain and plays an essential role in the existence and functioning of brain neurons involved in the development of motivation, attention, arousal as well as memory and cognition. The increased levels of NGF are proven to boost memory and enhance learning.

Research suggests that the Lion's Mane can be a potent neuroprotective, which could prove useful to treat a range of diseases, such as damage to the liver or obesity. It could also be helpful in treating certain types of cancer.

Chapter 14: Benefits And Effects

One of the most thrilling features that is unique to Lion's Mane is that it dramatically increases the levels of the nerve growth factor (NGF) that is a distinct kind of brain protein that has a crucial role to play in neuroplasticity, learning, and memory.

A high level of NGF are linked to optimal performance, brain health and resiliency. NGF shields neurons in the present and plays a crucial role in the process of neurogenesis, which is the regeneration of neural connections that are damaged by age, injury or disease. Lion's Mane has also demonstrated significant antioxidant and anti-inflammatory qualities that add to its neuroprotective capabilities.

The typical dosage ranges between 500 and 3000 mg daily.

Most often, the adverse effect of the condition is a rash on the skin that could be attributed to increasing the level of nerve growth factor. This indicates that you're healing but isn't an itching as a result of allergy or poisoning.

Though it's not listed It also regulates A1C. It can be a test which provides a picture of how your blood sugar is over the past three or two months. the majority of diabetics are aware and, even if they are on medication that regulates blood sugar, they always see very high levels. It is my belief that it controls it since I know a person who has diabetes who suffers from polyneuropathy. I advised the lion's horn for her, and it the results were not just better but also improved the quality of her life and quality of life, but I was also amazed to find that the results of the A1C was normal range after using the lion's Mane for 3 months. Her doctor was pleased with the results. In the same time frame, someone close to me had a stroke, and was diagnosed in the hospital where had diabetes. I mentioned my friend and he took it on, but the last test result for A1C was 8.0 After having taken lion's mane for 6 months, he retested the test once more and came back with the score of 5.9.

It's not a random event. In the case of neuropathic signs, you'll begin to see changes after the third or the fourth week of using the medication daily.

I suggest starting by taking 1 gram of the lion's Mane powder. It is packaged with a teaspoon which is a measure of the quantity of one milligram. The initial two weeks, you'll use 2 grams of it, which amounts to two teaspoons daily Then you will take one teaspoon daily or mix it into milk or juices, but I would not suggest mixing drinking it in water as the flavor isn't very appealing. After you have finished the powder you can purchase it as pills be sure to ensure it's natural, with no other additives and contains one thousand mg or one gram which is exactly the same. The lion's mane powder is one I'd like to have for the rest of my daily use because it can prevent Parkinson's and Alzheimer's. It can be consumed anytime of the day.

Below, I'll present the amino acids and antioxidants I consider vital, and when combined with the B-complex vitamins helped me to recover myelin that was destroyed and repaired the nervous system.

Glutathione:

It's a protein is produced naturally by us and whose primary function is to safeguard every cell tissue and organs which are part of our body. It's composed of 3 amino acids which are known as glutamate, glycine and cysteine. They are located in every one cell. The combination of these three amino acids creates the strongest antioxidant found in the body. In fact, some researchers consider it to be the "master antioxidant".. Antioxidants are essential for eliminating free radicals out of your body. Free radicals are fundamentally aggressive particles that strike every cell, harming all they come into contact with.

Glutathione's primary purpose is to shield mitochondria and cells from damage caused by free radicals, peroxidation and oxidation.

The problems that arise as we get older, which is because aging also impacts the capacity of our bodies to make glutathione.

The presence of low levels of glutathione is often linked to certain neurodegenerative conditions including Lou Gehrig's disease muscular atrophy or Parkinson's or Alzheimer's disease. which affects our Central Nervous System. Glutathione serves as a protection agent against xenobiotic poisoning, i.e. it guards against harm caused by the usage of drugs, medications pollution, carcinogens and environmental contaminants.

Many foods are rich in glutathione. Yet, regardless of foods that have glutathione as a component there are some who should look to supplements since the numerous causes reduce the amount of this protein within the body. This increases the risk of contracting illnesses previously unaffected. Smoking, stress as well as infections from intense sport exercise or environmental pollutants are just a few examples of the causes.

The problem is that glutathione can't be absorption when it is taken orally therefore, these supplements are nearly useless. It is feasible to increase the levels of glutathione in your body while using other supplements like vitamin C, cysteine Lipoic Acid, and N-Acetylcysteine.

N-acetylcysteine (NAC):

It's an acetylated variant of cysteine, an amino acid. It has a high antioxidant power due to having a thiol component. It is extremely stable and can be employed to lower the oxidative stress.

In the human body, N-Acetyl Cysteine is transformed to the antioxidant glutathione. At first, N-Acetyl cysteine transforms to cysteine, and the glutathione levels increase. N-Acetyl Cystine can travel through cell membranes and have an effect in the interior of the cell. It also maintains the levels of glutathione in cells that are high, which reduces the active oxygen species as well as oxygen-induced stress.

N-Acetyl Cysteine is a potent antioxidant as well as a cellular detoxifier. It helps neutralize free radicals as well being able to eliminate and block poisonous heavy metals, such as lead, mercury and Cadmium.

N-Acetyl Cysteine stabilizes the protein structure and helps in the formation of collagen.

Dose:

A ergogenic supplement, for ergogenic purposes, the daily dosage is approximately 20 mg/kg/day, broken down into doses of around 600 mg.

It is suggested to take N-Acetyl Cysteine with a full stomach as a result of its effects of chelation, it could lower the bioavailability for certain minerals. Because of this, it is suggested to consume these shots no less than 2 hours before or immediately after meals. Also, it is recommended that you take plenty of fluids throughout your day.

alpha lipoic acid

It's also known as ALA it is also referred to as thioctic or lipoic acid.

It's a potent antioxidant, and also functions as a cofactor in mitochondrial reactions where glucose is transformed into energy.

The efficiency of lipoic acids has been demonstrated in numerous studies on people with type 2 diabetes and excellent outcomes have been achieved. Alongside its effect on blood sugar levels, ALA is a shield against damage to renal vessels and reduces the symptoms of neuropathy and enhances the function of nerves. There is a strong belief that the reason for its significant role for protecting nerve cells comes from its ability to dissolve in water and fat. This allows you to access difficult nerve tissues and shield the nerve cells from peroxidation.

Alpha lipoic acid is a neuroprotective qualities. The studies of patients suffering from Alzheimer's, Parkinson's or other mental disorders have shown that decreasing oxidative stress within the nervous system can reduce the extent of damage and severity of the conditions. The study suggests that it can even slow the loss of memory caused by age, and also protects the brain against certain poisons.

It's also been proven that it is effective in protecting the nervous system in the event of traumatic injury. In the event of such injury it is known that inflammatory and oxidative destruction of nerve cells is enhanced and the alpha-lipoic acid intake has been proven to minimize the harm caused by these conditions.

Primary bodily functions:

As an antioxidant, it also acts as a neutralizes free radicals.

Protect against diabetic neuropathy.

Increase insulin response through reducing the amount of glucose that is present in blood.

The translocation of GLUT4 sugar transporters into cells' membranes.

The adipocytes are able to increase the amount of glucose that they absorb as well as muscle cells.

Improve blood flow to nerve ends.

It acts as a neuroprotective neural regeneration agent.

Improve cognitive function by stabilizing the brain and improving memory.

Improve the cerebral blood flow.

Invoke intracellular signaling pathways that can increase the longevity of neurons helping to treat cases of Alzheimer's Parkinson's, Parkinson's and similar neurological diseases that result from the oxidative process, inadequate blood supply, and the excessive demise of neurons.

Increase the capacity for detoxification of the liver.

The increase in glutathione levels.

Improve the immune response.

Reducing levels of triglycerides and high density lipoproteins.

Encourage the conversion of carbs to energy.

Dose:

The use of it as an antioxidant for healthy individuals is typically 50 to 100 mg. People with diabetes generally take 100-200 mg three times daily while you are taking therapeutic doses, the amount employed is much higher, and falls between 1600 and 1800 mg/day.

Lysine:

It is a vital amino acid, which has antioxidant power and is an essential ingredient in proteins. It is therefore essential in the development of muscles, the healing of wounded and injured areas, as well as the creation of enzymes, hormones and antibodies, and aids in the creation of collagen as well as healing of tissue. It is also involved in calcium absorption, and also stimulates the release of the growth hormone.

Lysine can be found in variety of foods. However, the main sources include:

Origins of animals Red cuts of meat, pork, poultry as well as fish (cod and Sardines) and cheese (especially Parmesan) and eggs.

Vegetables are the source of this. Although at lower levels than the meat industry, lysine can be present in brewer's yeast legumes and whole grains, seeds, carob as well as asparagus, watercress as well as spinach.

Dose:

Dietary requirements vary from 800 to 3000 mg/day.

The typical dose is 500 to 1,000 mg/day.

To ensure better absorption, it's best to consume the supplement with a full stomach. Furthermore Vitamin B6 helps in absorption.

Precautions:

Consuming lysine is usually very secure. doses of as little as three grams daily of lysine are easily tolerated. High doses of more than 15 grams per day, can trigger gastrointestinal discomfort, such as stomach cramps, nausea or diarrhea.

Lysine supplementation should not be considered for people suffering from hyperlysinemia or hyperlysinuria. Individuals with kidney or liver ailments should not consume Lysine supplements without the guidance of a medical professional.

Chapter 15: The Proline

Proline is among the amino acids that form made up of protein. Proline is made by glutamic acid directly which is why it's not an essential amino acid.

Proline is a key component of the production of collagen and due to this reason it is vital for restoration, healing and maintaining of a variety of tissues like connective, bone and muscle. Additionally, it's involved in the formation of ligaments and tendons.

Proline can be used as a treatment aid for treatment of joint problems due to its role in the process of collagen synthesizing. The most common cases are sprains and arthritis or injury to the ligament, lumbago tendinitis, dislocations and torticollis.

In addition, because of its participation in collagen synthesis, it's employed to improve the texture of the skin, and lessen the appearance of age, assist in the healing process of burns, wounds, and ulcers and as a cardioprotector in preventing arterial collagen from breaking down.

Proline can be found in foods.

Origins of animal, including fish, meat dairy, eggs and other animal products.

It is also found in foods.

Origins like seeds, legumes whole grains, fruit as well as nuts and other vegetables that are high in vitamin C.

Dose:

Since it's not an essential amino acid, there's not any publicly available data regarding the daily demands. The dosage as a diet supplement usually is close to 500 mg.

Precautions:

Proline is usually considered to be safe. In the event that people with kidney and liver problems shouldn't consume large quantities of amino acids without supervision of a qualified medical professional it is important to be aware of the fact that proline consumption can boost the quantity of amino acids that they consume throughout the throughout the day.

Histidine:

It is regarded as an amino acid that is semi-essential because adults produce it in adequate quantity, but children do not. Histidine is used by our body for making proteins and enzymes as well as the production of histamine.

A few of the advantages of histidine include:

Histidine plays a role in immediate as well as allergic hypersensitivity reactions.

One of the major advantages of histidine is that it assists in the elimination of heavy metals out of the body.

It helps in the development and healing of tissues. essential to recover myelin.

Essential in the development of white and red blood cells.

It is anti-inflammatory and has properties.

One of the other properties and advantages of histidine is that it aids in improving digestion, as it increases in the creation of stomach juices.

The other benefit of histidine is the fact that it helps strengthen the system of immigration

They're a great source of histidine

Beef, lamb and pork as well as their derivatives.

Fish, chicken, as well as dairy items.

A high level of histidine are harmful, and having low levels of it contributes to the rheumatoid arthritis

Take a supplement of histidine along with vitamin

Vitamin B6 and B3 converts it to histamine.

Histamine is a natural ingredient found in Rye, wheat, and rice.

Like I've said in the past that the nervous system is regenerated every 8 months, and in order to replenish it, it needs the following minerals and vitamins:

Vitamin B12

Folic Acid

Vitamin B6

Vitamin B1

Vitamin B3 Niacin(not the form of niacidin sold as B3)

Magnesium

Potassium

These are the most crucial of them, and if you do not have one, you will not properly regenerate. Magnesium, a mineral which about 90 percent of people suffer from deficiency and is among the main causes of neuropathy however, no physician has mentioned this issue, or even the physicians who have helped me. Potassium functions in tandem with magnesium. The two together aid in the elimination of sodium excess out of the body. There are a variety of magnesium. However, after a lot of research, I settled on magnesium glycinate due to the fact that glycine, an amino acid that is very relaxing boosts immune cells which aid in cleaning the damaged or damaged tissue. Additionally, it aids in the creation of Collagen. Magnesium Glycinate aids in relaxing in the evening and alleviates joint or muscle pain that you experience during the night.

In contrast you will find the elements which affect the nervous system, and can overload it. Therefore, it's crucial to remove those triggers or at a minimum, the ones that you can eliminate, since the environmental and wifi pollution are something that cannot be changed but it affects the nervous system. However, this is where glutathione can come in to play an important function. We can't alter the world, but if could increase our levels glutathione, that's what's protecting and defending our bodies. For me, the most efficient way to increase glutathione levels is to take alpha lipoic acid, acetylcysteine, and vitamin C of 1000 mg.

Other elements that impact the nervous system are:

*The presence of chemicals in processed foods

Some medications include antibiotics, antacids and anticonvulsants etc. If I'm given an antibiotic or other drug that I am prescribed, the first thing I check for any adverse reactions to ensure that it's not affecting the nervous system. If it does, I inform my doctor to switch it with a different one.

Stress, we are aware of the dangers as stress build over the entire central nervous system. Eventually, eventually, excessive stress overburdens the nervous system. Just as the electrical cables which become overloaded. When they are heated, they get hot and cause the rubber to melt which covers the cable. which is how it occurs with nerves. Then, it is lost the myelin which protects it. Then, there is neuropathy. This is the reason it's crucial to know how to reduce stress. And when we do experience it, be aware of the best way to release it in a way that it will not build up inside our bodies and negatively impact our health.